SEVEN PILLARS

OF FREEDOM

JOURNAL

SEVEN PILLARS OF FREEDOM JOURNAL

Published by
Pure Desire Ministries International
719 NE Roberts Avenue, Gresham, OR 97030
www.puredesire.org | 503.489.0230
ISBN 978-1-943291-89-2

2nd Edition with revisions, September 2021

Content editing by Heather Kolb

Cover design, interior design, and typesetting by Elisabeth Windsor

THIS BOOK BELONGS TO

_____

GROUP MEMBERS

Name _____   Number _____

Name _____   Number _____

Name _____   Number _____

Name _____   Number _____

Name _____   Number _____

CONTENTS

WELCOME TO THE JOURNEY

I'm sure you have heard the famous quote by theologian Lynn H. Hough, "The joy is in the journey not the destination." Although I did not recognize it at the time, looking back now at my experience in Seven Pillars groups over the years, I agree with Hough. Being a goal-driven workaholic, I so desperately wanted to learn all of the information the workbook could render, apply the truths to my life, and find freedom from bondage as quickly as possible.

This is how the typical addict thinks: *the people around me have noticed my flaws. Let's figure out what's wrong, patch the holes, and keep moving.*

As you can imagine (or may have already experienced), this approach to healing simply doesn't work. Change is not free or easy; it always costs you something. If you have read any Pure Desire resources or been to a Pure Desire event, you have probably heard the phrase, "Trying harder doesn't work." That doesn't mean the work you are about to embark on in *Seven Pillars of Freedom* will be easy. If done correctly, this work will be some of the most emotionally, mentally, and spiritually challenging you have ever completed. "Trying harder" is about trying to look good and keep it together. The hard work in this study is about evaluating how you see yourself, the important people in your life, and God, and how you believe God sees you. It's a daily process of spending more time and energy on your healing than the time and energy you used to invest in your addiction.

The purpose of this journal is to reinforce the daily commitment to health, which we refer to as self care. Self care is vital to your sobriety, as well as your spiritual growth. It is imperative that you are investing in your recovery every day. On the following pages, you will find a list of the tools provided in this journal to help you develop this daily discipline.

COMMITMENT TO CHANGE

This addresses a challenge you will be facing during the week or a behavior you have identified that needs to change. This Commitment to Change is about something you have identified that will help you move forward in your restoration. Fill out the Commitment to Change in your group time and evaluate the Double Bind (what you have to give up to make this change).

VIDEO COMPANION

Navigating your healing journey can be challenging. Throughout this group, we want to equip you with all of the tools you need to bring your best effort to each lesson. For this reason, we have created a companion video for every lesson in this group, including the introduction and the conclusion. Watching these videos will help you have a great, life-changing group experience! Be sure to watch these videos during the week before you begin working through the lesson, as you will hear helpful insights and tips on that lesson from our Executive Director, Nick Stumbo. Each video is about 4-5 minutes in length. You can access these videos any time by logging in to your account at puredesire.org/courses.

 Watch the two videos under "Start Here" in the Video Companion (*Introduction* and *The Tools*) before starting group.

DEVOTIONAL

The battlefield for purity is totally in your mind. Paul declares in Romans 12:2 that transformation is a process of renewing the mind. This is why it is so important that you are spending time in God's Word. In this journal we have included a weekly study of the book of Proverbs. If you have a daily reading plan, take one day each week and spend your devotional time with your Pure Desire group in Proverbs. If you don't regularly read your Bible, use this opportunity to start reading it at least once a week.

FASTER SCALE

You need to choose at least three days each week when you will commit to calling another group member. Before each call, review the FASTER Scale and identify how far down the scale you have moved since the last call or group meeting, based on the emotions and behaviors you have experienced. During your call, answer the following three questions relating to where you are at on the FASTER Scale, plus the two follow-up questions:

FASTER SCALE:

+ How does it affect you? How do you act/feel?
+ How does it affect the important people in your life?
+ Why do you do this? What is the benefit for you?

FOLLOW-UP:

+ What do you need to do to get back to restoration?
+ How are you doing on your Commitment to Change?

GROUP CHECK-IN

This questionnaire will help you evaluate the patterns you identified on the FASTER Scale, progress you have made on your Commitment to Change, and progress you're making in the important relationships in your life each week.

Spend at least thirty minutes each day working through the homework, making calls, reading the weekly devotional, evaluating your FASTER Scale, or completing your Group Check-in. Below is an example schedule for completing the work in a typical week.

Tuesday	+ Went to group
Wednesday	+ Watched the Video Companion and completed the reading for Pillar Two: Lesson Three
Thursday	+ Worked through the FASTER Scale, called Joe to talk about the Double Bind related to Speeding Up
Friday	+ Read the Devotional, completed the SWORD Drill
Saturday	+ Worked through the FASTER Scale, called Steve, answered the questions in Lesson Three
Sunday	+ Worked through the FASTER Scale, called Tim, finished Lesson Three homework
Monday	+ Filled out the Group Check-in

This process will be challenging; it will require time and energy to do well. Our prayer is that you will find the journey worthwhile. A life free from addiction is a great blessing, but the journey of spiritual and emotional growth is an even greater reward.

SWORD DRILL

LEARN TO JOURNAL IN RESPONSE TO THE WORD OF GOD

Practice the SWORD Drill throughout your time in this workbook. Otherwise the truths you discover will not be tied to Scripture and will lack transformational power. In other words, you will be touched but unchanged. This process involves some of the most significant renewing of your mind you have ever experienced and that only happens when you encounter the supernatural power of God's Word in your heart and not just in your head.

Through the years I have found the term SWORD to be very helpful in the journaling process. It reminds me that this is about spiritual warfare. This isn't just about some clinical process; this is WAR. I need to approach each day of the rest of my life with the weapon of the Word of God in my heart and on my mouth.

SWORD (SCRIPTURE. WAIT. OBSERVE. REQUEST. DEDICATE.)

S - SCRIPTURE

You will learn many great neurological and psychological truths in this workbook. But real change in your direction in life only comes from the Word of God. This life is just the introductory page to eternity. You will live with the character you develop in this short life here on earth. In fact, you only take two things out of this world: character and relationships. And apart from the grace of God and the wisdom of His Word you will mess up on both accounts. God's Word is the hope of my heart; it speaks renewed hope when I have given up on myself and gives courage to my soul when I am facing overwhelming odds.

W - WAIT

I have done the daily scripture readings through the Bible, and over the long haul they leave me hollow. I am so busy reading through the required passages to get through the Bible in a year that it becomes another frantic thing I do in my busy life. The Benedictine tradition of Lectio Divina gets it right; it is the ancient practice of reading scripture meditatively—not to master the Word, not to criticize the Word, but to be mastered and challenged by the Word. It is the process of allowing the Word to read and interpret us.

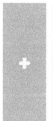

Give this a try—first read the passage on your knees.
Read it aloud, slowly, attentively. Then pause to let it sink in. Read the passage aloud again, this time asking the question, "Where am I in the passage?" Finally, read the passage again noticing what word or words jump out at you, grabbing your attention. Meditate on those words. Chew on them for a while.

O - OBSERVE

Writing down what you observe clarifies the thought processes and involves another whole section of your brain. Now have a seat and read the passage with pencil in hand and note what you have observed.

R - REQUEST THAT THE HOLY SPIRIT HELP YOU SEE HOW ALL OF THIS APPLIES TO YOUR LIFE

This is not an academic process but a process of the heart. You are specifically asking the Word to read you. This is a supernatural process that frequently triggers a neurochemical cascade of new understanding where your mind is being renewed.

D - DEDICATE YOURSELF

The one thing that moves us from being just touched by God to truly being changed is the commitment of our heart and will. Trying harder will never get us headed in the right direction when it comes to getting free from our sexual struggles. But once the Holy Spirit gets us headed in the right direction, dedicating ourselves to that direction in life will change us.

PILLAR ONE
LESSON ONE

DIRECTION DETERMINES DESTINATION
WORKBOOK PAGE / 30

☐ The Tools Video

☐ Seven Pillars Intro Video

☐ Pillar One Intro Video

☐ Pillar One: Lesson One Video

☐ Workbook Assignment

☐ *Pure Desire* Reading

☐ Commitment to Change

☐ Devotional

☐ FASTER Scale

☐ Group Check-in

➕ **Read Chapter 1 in *Pure Desire*. What were your observations?**

COMMITMENT TO CHANGE

1   What area do you need to change or what challenge are you facing next week?

2   What will it cost you emotionally if you do change? What fear will you have to face?

3   What will it cost you if you don't change?

4   What is your plan to maintain your restoration regarding these changes?

5   Who will you be accountable to as you pursue this commitment?

6   What are the details of this commitment? What information will you share with your accountability team when you touch base with them this week?

DEVOTIONAL

²¹ With persuasive words she led him astray;
she seduced him with her smooth talk.
²² All at once he followed her
like an ox going to the slaughter,
like a deer stepping into a noose
²³ till an arrow pierces his liver,
like a bird darting into a snare,
little knowing it will cost him his life.

²⁴ Now then, my sons, listen to me;
pay attention to what I say.
²⁵ Do not let your heart turn to her ways
or stray into her paths.
²⁶ Many are the victims she has brought down;
her slain are a mighty throng.
²⁷ Her house is a highway to the grave,
leading down to the chambers of death.

PROVERBS 7:21-27

 Read Proverbs 7.

SWORD DRILL

 S **cripture** - Which verse or group of verses stood out to you in the Proverbs reading? Write it/them below.

 W **ait** - Take a few moments now to wait on the Holy Spirit. Put aside any thoughts and worries of the day. Meditate on the Scripture. Read the verse(s) above aloud, slowly and attentively. Then pause to let it sink in. Let the Holy Spirit speak to you.

 O **bserve** - What did you notice about the verse(s) from above? Was there something that the Holy Spirit spoke to you? Write your observation below.

 R **equest** - Ask God to show you where and how the Scripture and observation apply to your life. Write the application below.

 D **edicate Yourself** - Looking at how the Scripture applies to you, what is one thing that needs to change? Remember, this is not necessarily about something you need to do (or stop doing). Perhaps the change is in the way you see yourself or others.

FASTER SCALE

Adapted with permission from *The Genesis Process* by Michael Dye.

- Circle the behaviors that you identify with in each section.
- Identify the most powerful behavior in each section and write it next to the corresponding heading.
- Answer the following three questions:
  1. How does it affect me? How do I feel in the moment?
  2. How does it affect the important people in my life?
  3. Why do I do this? What is the benefit for me?

RESTORATION _____

(Accepting life on God's terms, with trust, grace, mercy, vulnerability and gratitude.) No current secrets; working to resolve problems; identifying fears and feelings; keeping commitments to meetings, prayer, family, church, people, goals, and self; being open and honest, making eye contact; increasing in relationships with God and others; true accountability.

1. _____
2. _____
3. _____

FORGETTING PRIORITIES _____

(Start believing the present circumstances and moving away from trusting God. Denial; flight; a change in what's important; how you spend your time, energy, and thoughts.) Secrets; less time/energy for God, meetings, church; avoiding support and accountability people; superficial conversations; sarcasm; isolating; changes in goals; obsessed with relationships; breaking promises and commitments; neglecting family; preoccupation with material things, TV, computers, entertainment; procrastination; lying; overconfidence; bored; hiding money; image management; seeking to control situations and other people.

1. _____
   _____
2. _____
   _____
3. _____
   _____

ANXIETY

(A growing background noise of undefined fear; getting energy from emotions.)
Worry, using profanity, being fearful; being resentful; replaying old, negative
thoughts; perfectionism; judging other's motives; making goals and lists that you
can't complete; mind reading; fantasy, codependent rescuing; sleep problems,
trouble concentrating, seeking/creating drama; gossip; using over-the-counter
medication for pain, sleep or weight control; flirting.

1. _____
   _____

2. _____
   _____

3. _____
   _____

SPEEDING UP

(Trying to outrun the anxiety which is usually the first sign of depression.) Super
busy and always in a hurry (finding good reason to justify the work); workaholic; can't
relax; avoiding slowing down; feeling driven; can't turn off thoughts; skipping meals;
binge eating (usually at night); overspending; can't identify own feelings/needs;
repetitive negative thoughts; irritable; dramatic mood swings; too much caffeine; over
exercising; nervousness; difficulty being alone and/or with people; difficulty listening
to others; making excuses for having to "do it all."

1. _____
   _____

2. _____
   _____

3. _____
   _____

TICKED OFF

(Getting adrenaline high on anger and aggression.) Procrastination causing crisis in
money, work, and relationships; increased sarcasm; black and white (all or nothing)
thinking; feeling alone; nobody understands; overreacting, road rage; constant resentments;
pushing others away; increasing isolation; blaming; arguing; irrational thinking; can't
take criticism; defensive; people avoiding you; needing to be right; digestive problems;
headaches; obsessive (stuck) thoughts; can't forgive; feeling superior; using intimidation.

1. _____

_____

2. _____

_____

3. _____

_____

EXHAUSTED _____

(Loss of physical and emotional energy; coming off the adrenaline high, and the onset of depression.) Depressed; panicked; confused; hopelessness; sleeping too much or too little; can't cope; overwhelmed; crying for "no reason"; can't think; forgetful; pessimistic; helpless; tired; numb; wanting to run; constant cravings for old coping behaviors; thinking of using sex, drugs, or alcohol; seeking old unhealthy people and places; really isolating; people angry with you; self abuse; suicidal thoughts; spontaneous crying; no goals; survival mode; not returning phone calls; missing work; irritability; no appetite.

1. _____

_____

2. _____

_____

3. _____

_____

RELAPSE _____

(Returning to the place you swore you would never go again. Coping with life on your terms. You sitting in the driver's seat instead of God.) Giving up and giving in; out of control; lost in your addiction; lying to yourself and others; feeling you just can't manage without your coping behaviors, at least for now. The result is the reinforcement of shame, guilt and condemnation; and feelings of abandonment and being alone.

1. _____

_____

2. _____

_____

3. _____

_____

GROUP CHECK-IN

COMPLETE 24 HOURS BEFORE GROUP

1 What is the lowest level you reached on the *FASTER Scale* this week?

2 What was the *Double Bind* you were dealing with?

3 Where are you on your *Commitment to Change* from our last meeting?

4 Have you lied to anyone this week either directly or indirectly?

5 What have you done to improve your relationship with your wife or other significant relationships this week?

PILLAR ONE
LESSON TWO

POINTS OF POWERLESSNESS
WORKBOOK PAGE / 41

- [ ] Pillar One: Lesson Two Video
- [ ] Workbook Assignment
- [ ] *Pure Desire* Reading
- [ ] Commitment to Change
- [ ] Devotional
- [ ] FASTER Scale
- [ ] Group Check-in

Read Chapter 2 in *Pure Desire*. What were your observations?

COMMITMENT TO CHANGE

1   What area do you need to change or what challenge are you facing next week?

2   What will it cost you emotionally if you do change? What fear will you have to face?

3   What will it cost you if you don't change?

4   What is your plan to maintain your restoration regarding these changes?

5   Who will you be accountable to as you pursue this commitment?

6   What are the details of this commitment? What information will you share with your accountability team when you touch base with them this week?

DEVOTIONAL

¹⁶ Whoever strays from the path of prudence
comes to rest in the company of the dead.

¹⁷ Whoever loves pleasure will become poor;
whoever loves wine and olive oil will never be rich.

¹⁸ The wicked become a ransom for the righteous,
and the unfaithful for the upright.

¹⁹ Better to live in a desert
than with a quarrelsome and nagging wife.

²⁰ The wise store up choice food and olive oil,
but fools gulp theirs down.

²¹ Whoever pursues righteousness and love
finds life, prosperity and honor.

²² One who is wise can go up against the city of the mighty
and pull down the stronghold in which they trust.

²³ Those who guard their mouths and their tongues
keep themselves from calamity.

PROVERBS 21:16-23

 Read Proverbs 21.

SWORD DRILL

S **cripture** - Which verse or group of verses stood out to you in the Proverbs reading? Write it/them below.

W **ait** - Take a few moments now to wait on the Holy Spirit. Put aside any thoughts and worries of the day. Meditate on the Scripture. Read the verse(s) above aloud, slowly and attentively. Then pause to let it sink in. Let the Holy Spirit speak to you.

O **bserve** - What did you notice about the verse(s) from above? Was there something that the Holy Spirit spoke to you? Write your observation below.

R **equest** - Ask God to show you where and how the Scripture and observation apply to your life. Write the application below.

D **edicate Yourself** - Looking at how the Scripture applies to you, what is one thing that needs to change? Remember, this is not necessarily about something you need to do (or stop doing). Perhaps the change is in the way you see yourself or others.

FASTER SCALE

Adapted with permission from *The Genesis Process* by Michael Dye.

- Circle the behaviors that you identify with in each section.
- Identify the most powerful behavior in each section and write it next to the corresponding heading.
- Answer the following three questions:
  1. How does it affect me? How do I feel in the moment?
  2. How does it affect the important people in my life?
  3. Why do I do this? What is the benefit for me?

RESTORATION _____

(Accepting life on God's terms, with trust, grace, mercy, vulnerability and gratitude.) No current secrets; working to resolve problems; identifying fears and feelings; keeping commitments to meetings, prayer, family, church, people, goals, and self; being open and honest, making eye contact; increasing in relationships with God and others; true accountability.

1. _____
2. _____
3. _____

FORGETTING PRIORITIES _____

(Start believing the present circumstances and moving away from trusting God. Denial; flight; a change in what's important; how you spend your time, energy, and thoughts.) Secrets; less time/energy for God, meetings, church; avoiding support and accountability people; superficial conversations; sarcasm; isolating; changes in goals; obsessed with relationships; breaking promises and commitments; neglecting family; preoccupation with material things, TV, computers, entertainment; procrastination; lying; overconfidence; bored; hiding money; image management; seeking to control situations and other people.

1. _____
   _____
2. _____
   _____
3. _____
   _____

ANXIETY

(A growing background noise of undefined fear; getting energy from emotions.) Worry, using profanity, being fearful; being resentful; replaying old, negative thoughts; perfectionism; judging other's motives; making goals and lists that you can't complete; mind reading; fantasy, codependent rescuing; sleep problems, trouble concentrating, seeking/creating drama; gossip; using over-the-counter medication for pain, sleep or weight control; flirting.

1. _____

_____

2. _____

_____

3. _____

_____

SPEEDING UP

(Trying to outrun the anxiety which is usually the first sign of depression.) Super busy and always in a hurry (finding good reason to justify the work); workaholic; can't relax; avoiding slowing down; feeling driven; can't turn off thoughts; skipping meals; binge eating (usually at night); overspending; can't identify own feelings/needs; repetitive negative thoughts; irritable; dramatic mood swings; too much caffeine; over exercising; nervousness; difficulty being alone and/or with people; difficulty listening to others; making excuses for having to "do it all."

1. _____

_____

2. _____

_____

3. _____

_____

TICKED OFF

(Getting adrenaline high on anger and aggression.) Procrastination causing crisis in money, work, and relationships; increased sarcasm; black and white (all or nothing) thinking; feeling alone; nobody understands; overreacting, road rage; constant resentments; pushing others away; increasing isolation; blaming; arguing; irrational thinking; can't take criticism; defensive; people avoiding you; needing to be right; digestive problems; headaches; obsessive (stuck) thoughts; can't forgive; feeling superior; using intimidation.

1. _____

_____

2. _____

_____

3. _____

_____

EXHAUSTED _____

(Loss of physical and emotional energy; coming off the adrenaline high, and the onset of depression.) Depressed; panicked; confused; hopelessness; sleeping too much or too little; can't cope; overwhelmed; crying for "no reason"; can't think; forgetful; pessimistic; helpless; tired; numb; wanting to run; constant cravings for old coping behaviors; thinking of using sex, drugs, or alcohol; seeking old unhealthy people and places; really isolating; people angry with you; self abuse; suicidal thoughts; spontaneous crying; no goals; survival mode; not returning phone calls; missing work; irritability; no appetite.

1. _____

_____

2. _____

_____

3. _____

_____

RELAPSE _____

(Returning to the place you swore you would never go again. Coping with life on your terms. You sitting in the driver's seat instead of God.) Giving up and giving in; out of control; lost in your addiction; lying to yourself and others; feeling you just can't manage without your coping behaviors, at least for now. The result is the reinforcement of shame, guilt and condemnation; and feelings of abandonment and being alone.

1. _____

_____

2. _____

_____

3. _____

_____

GROUP CHECK-IN

COMPLETE 24 HOURS BEFORE GROUP

1   What is the lowest level you reached on the *FASTER Scale* this week?

2   What was the *Double Bind* you were dealing with?

3   Where are you on your *Commitment to Change* from our last meeting?

4   Have you lied to anyone this week either directly or indirectly?

5   What have you done to improve your relationship with your wife or other significant relationships this week?

PILLAR ONE
LESSON THREE

EXITING THE HIGHWAY OF DENIAL
WORKBOOK PAGE / 47

☐ Pillar One: Lesson Three Video

☐ Workbook Assignment

☐ Commitment to Change

☐ Devotional

☐ FASTER Scale

☐ Group Check-in

COMMITMENT TO CHANGE

1   What area do you need to change or what challenge are you facing next week?

2   What will it cost you emotionally if you do change? What fear will you have to face?

3   What will it cost you if you don't change?

4   What is your plan to maintain your restoration regarding these changes?

5   Who will you be accountable to as you pursue this commitment?

6   What are the details of this commitment? What information will you share with your accountability team when you touch base with them this week?

DEVOTIONAL

Wisdom has built her house;
she has set up its seven pillars.
² She has prepared her meat and mixed her wine;
she has also set her table.
³ She has sent out her servants, and she calls
from the highest point of the city,
⁴ "Let all who are simple come to my house!"
To those who have no sense she says,
⁵ "Come, eat my food
and drink the wine I have mixed.
⁶ Leave your simple ways and you will live;
walk in the way of insight."

⁷ Whoever corrects a mocker invites insults;
whoever rebukes the wicked incurs abuse.
⁸ Do not rebuke mockers or they will hate you;
rebuke the wise and they will love you.

PROVERBS 9:1-8

 Read Proverbs 9.

SWORD DRILL

S **cripture** - Which verse or group of verses stood out to you in the Proverbs reading? Write it/them below.

W **ait** - Take a few moments now to wait on the Holy Spirit. Put aside any thoughts and worries of the day. Meditate on the Scripture. Read the verse(s) above aloud, slowly and attentively. Then pause to let it sink in. Let the Holy Spirit speak to you.

O **bserve** - What did you notice about the verse(s) from above? Was there something that the Holy Spirit spoke to you? Write your observation below.

R **equest** - Ask God to show you where and how the Scripture and observation apply to your life. Write the application below.

D **edicate Yourself** - Looking at how the Scripture applies to you, what is one thing that needs to change? Remember, this is not necessarily about something you need to do (or stop doing). Perhaps the change is in the way you see yourself or others.

FASTER SCALE

Adapted with permission from *The Genesis Process* by Michael Dye.

- Circle the behaviors that you identify with in each section.
- Identify the most powerful behavior in each section and write it next to the corresponding heading.
- Answer the following three questions:
  1. How does it affect me? How do I feel in the moment?
  2. How does it affect the important people in my life?
  3. Why do I do this? What is the benefit for me?

RESTORATION _____

(Accepting life on God's terms, with trust, grace, mercy, vulnerability and gratitude.) No current secrets; working to resolve problems; identifying fears and feelings; keeping commitments to meetings, prayer, family, church, people, goals, and self; being open and honest, making eye contact; increasing in relationships with God and others; true accountability.

1. _____
2. _____
3. _____

FORGETTING PRIORITIES _____

(Start believing the present circumstances and moving away from trusting God. Denial; flight; a change in what's important; how you spend your time, energy, and thoughts.) Secrets; less time/energy for God, meetings, church; avoiding support and accountability people; superficial conversations; sarcasm; isolating; changes in goals; obsessed with relationships; breaking promises and commitments; neglecting family; preoccupation with material things, TV, computers, entertainment; procrastination; lying; overconfidence; bored; hiding money; image management; seeking to control situations and other people.

1. _____
   _____
2. _____
   _____
3. _____
   _____

ANXIETY

(A growing background noise of undefined fear; getting energy from emotions.) Worry, using profanity, being fearful; being resentful; replaying old, negative thoughts; perfectionism; judging other's motives; making goals and lists that you can't complete; mind reading; fantasy, codependent rescuing; sleep problems, trouble concentrating, seeking/creating drama; gossip; using over-the-counter medication for pain, sleep or weight control; flirting.

1. _____
   _____

2. _____
   _____

3. _____
   _____

SPEEDING UP

(Trying to outrun the anxiety which is usually the first sign of depression.) Super busy and always in a hurry (finding good reason to justify the work); workaholic; can't relax; avoiding slowing down; feeling driven; can't turn off thoughts; skipping meals; binge eating (usually at night); overspending; can't identify own feelings/needs; repetitive negative thoughts; irritable; dramatic mood swings; too much caffeine; over exercising; nervousness; difficulty being alone and/or with people; difficulty listening to others; making excuses for having to "do it all."

1. _____
   _____

2. _____
   _____

3. _____
   _____

TICKED OFF

(Getting adrenaline high on anger and aggression.) Procrastination causing crisis in money, work, and relationships; increased sarcasm; black and white (all or nothing) thinking; feeling alone; nobody understands; overreacting, road rage; constant resentments; pushing others away; increasing isolation; blaming; arguing; irrational thinking; can't take criticism; defensive; people avoiding you; needing to be right; digestive problems; headaches; obsessive (stuck) thoughts; can't forgive; feeling superior; using intimidation.

1. _____

2. _____

3. _____

EXHAUSTED _____

(Loss of physical and emotional energy; coming off the adrenaline high, and the onset of depression.) Depressed; panicked; confused; hopelessness; sleeping too much or too little; can't cope; overwhelmed; crying for "no reason"; can't think; forgetful; pessimistic; helpless; tired; numb; wanting to run; constant cravings for old coping behaviors; thinking of using sex, drugs, or alcohol; seeking old unhealthy people and places; really isolating; people angry with you; self abuse; suicidal thoughts; spontaneous crying; no goals; survival mode; not returning phone calls; missing work; irritability; no appetite.

1. _____

2. _____

3. _____

RELAPSE _____

(Returning to the place you swore you would never go again. Coping with life on your terms. You sitting in the driver's seat instead of God.) Giving up and giving in; out of control; lost in your addiction; lying to yourself and others; feeling you just can't manage without your coping behaviors, at least for now. The result is the reinforcement of shame, guilt and condemnation; and feelings of abandonment and being alone.

1. _____

2. _____

3. _____

GROUP CHECK-IN

COMPLETE 24 HOURS BEFORE GROUP

1 What is the lowest level you reached on the *FASTER Scale* this week?

2 What was the *Double Bind* you were dealing with?

3 Where are you on your *Commitment to Change* from our last meeting?

4 Have you lied to anyone this week either directly or indirectly?

5 What have you done to improve your relationship with your wife or other significant relationships this week?

PILLAR ONE
LESSON FOUR

THE ROAD TO RECOVERY
WORKBOOK PAGE / 55

+ **Read Chapters 3 and 4 in *Pure Desire*. What were your observations?**

COMMITMENT TO CHANGE

1   What area do you need to change or what challenge are you facing next week?

2   What will it cost you emotionally if you do change? What fear will you have to face?

3   What will it cost you if you don't change?

4   What is your plan to maintain your restoration regarding these changes?

5   Who will you be accountable to as you pursue this commitment?

6   What are the details of this commitment? What information will you share with your accountability team when you touch base with them this week?

DEVOTIONAL

My son, do not forget my teaching,
but keep my commands in your heart,
² for they will prolong your life many years
and bring you peace and prosperity.

³ Let love and faithfulness never leave you;
bind them around your neck,
write them on the tablet of your heart.
⁴ Then you will win favor and a good name
in the sight of God and man.

⁵ Trust in the Lord with all your heart
and lean not on your own understanding;
⁶ in all your ways submit to him,
and he will make your paths straight.

⁷ Do not be wise in your own eyes;
fear the Lord and shun evil.
⁸ This will bring health to your body
and nourishment to your bones.

PROVERBS 3:1-8

 Read Proverbs 3.

SWORD DRILL

Scripture - Which verse or group of verses stood out to you in the Proverbs reading? Write it/them below.

Wait - Take a few moments now to wait on the Holy Spirit. Put aside any thoughts and worries of the day. Meditate on the Scripture. Read the verse(s) above aloud, slowly and attentively. Then pause to let it sink in. Let the Holy Spirit speak to you.

Observe - What did you notice about the verse(s) from above? Was there something that the Holy Spirit spoke to you? Write your observation below.

Request - Ask God to show you where and how the Scripture and observation apply to your life. Write the application below.

Dedicate Yourself - Looking at how the Scripture applies to you, what is one thing that needs to change? Remember, this is not necessarily about something you need to do (or stop doing). Perhaps the change is in the way you see yourself or others.

FASTER SCALE

Adapted with permission from *The Genesis Process* by Michael Dye.

- ✦ **Circle the behaviors that you identify with in each section.**
- ✦ **Identify the most powerful behavior in each section and write it next to the corresponding heading.**
- ✦ **Answer the following three questions:**
  1. How does it affect me? How do I feel in the moment?
  2. How does it affect the important people in my life?
  3. Why do I do this? What is the benefit for me?

RESTORATION _____

(Accepting life on God's terms, with trust, grace, mercy, vulnerability and gratitude.) No current secrets; working to resolve problems; identifying fears and feelings; keeping commitments to meetings, prayer, family, church, people, goals, and self; being open and honest, making eye contact; increasing in relationships with God and others; true accountability.

1. _____
2. _____
3. _____

FORGETTING PRIORITIES _____

(Start believing the present circumstances and moving away from trusting God. Denial; flight; a change in what's important; how you spend your time, energy, and thoughts.) Secrets; less time/energy for God, meetings, church; avoiding support and accountability people; superficial conversations; sarcasm; isolating; changes in goals; obsessed with relationships; breaking promises and commitments; neglecting family; preoccupation with material things, TV, computers, entertainment; procrastination; lying; overconfidence; bored; hiding money; image management; seeking to control situations and other people.

1. _____
   _____
2. _____
   _____
3. _____
   _____

ANXIETY

(A growing background noise of undefined fear; getting energy from emotions.)
Worry, using profanity, being fearful; being resentful; replaying old, negative
thoughts; perfectionism; judging other's motives; making goals and lists that you
can't complete; mind reading; fantasy, codependent rescuing; sleep problems,
trouble concentrating, seeking/creating drama; gossip; using over-the-counter
medication for pain, sleep or weight control; flirting.

1. _____

_____

2. _____

_____

3. _____

_____

SPEEDING UP

(Trying to outrun the anxiety which is usually the first sign of depression.) Super
busy and always in a hurry (finding good reason to justify the work); workaholic; can't
relax; avoiding slowing down; feeling driven; can't turn off thoughts; skipping meals;
binge eating (usually at night); overspending; can't identify own feelings/needs;
repetitive negative thoughts; irritable; dramatic mood swings; too much caffeine; over
exercising; nervousness; difficulty being alone and/or with people; difficulty listening
to others; making excuses for having to "do it all."

1. _____

_____

2. _____

_____

3. _____

_____

TICKED OFF

(Getting adrenaline high on anger and aggression.) Procrastination causing crisis in
money, work, and relationships; increased sarcasm; black and white (all or nothing)
thinking; feeling alone; nobody understands; overreacting, road rage; constant resentments;
pushing others away; increasing isolation; blaming; arguing; irrational thinking; can't
take criticism; defensive; people avoiding you; needing to be right; digestive problems;
headaches; obsessive (stuck) thoughts; can't forgive; feeling superior; using intimidation.

1. _____

2. _____

3. _____

EXHAUSTED _____

(Loss of physical and emotional energy; coming off the adrenaline high, and the onset of depression.) Depressed; panicked; confused; hopelessness; sleeping too much or too little; can't cope; overwhelmed; crying for "no reason"; can't think; forgetful; pessimistic; helpless; tired; numb; wanting to run; constant cravings for old coping behaviors; thinking of using sex, drugs, or alcohol; seeking old unhealthy people and places; really isolating; people angry with you; self abuse; suicidal thoughts; spontaneous crying; no goals; survival mode; not returning phone calls; missing work; irritability; no appetite.

1. _____

2. _____

3. _____

RELAPSE _____

(Returning to the place you swore you would never go again. Coping with life on your terms. You sitting in the driver's seat instead of God.) Giving up and giving in; out of control; lost in your addiction; lying to yourself and others; feeling you just can't manage without your coping behaviors, at least for now. The result is the reinforcement of shame, guilt and condemnation; and feelings of abandonment and being alone.

1. _____

2. _____

3. _____

GROUP CHECK-IN

COMPLETE 24 HOURS BEFORE GROUP

1   What is the lowest level you reached on the *FASTER Scale* this week?

2   What was the *Double Bind* you were dealing with?

3   Where are you on your *Commitment to Change* from our last meeting?

4   Have you lied to anyone this week either directly or indirectly?

5   What have you done to improve your relationship with your wife or other significant relationships this week?

PILLAR TWO
LESSON ONE

HOPE IN THE MIDST OF HOPELESSNESS
WORKBOOK PAGE / 64

☐ Pillar Two Intro Video

☐ Pillar Two: Lesson One Video

☐ Workbook Assignment

☐ *Pure Desire* Reading

☐ Commitment to Change

☐ Devotional

☐ FASTER Scale

☐ Group Check-in

+   **Read Chapter 5 in *Pure Desire*. What were your observations?**

COMMITMENT TO CHANGE

1 What area do you need to change or what challenge are you facing next week?

2 What will it cost you emotionally if you do change? What fear will you have to face?

3 What will it cost you if you don't change?

4 What is your plan to maintain your restoration regarding these changes?

5 Who will you be accountable to as you pursue this commitment?

6 What are the details of this commitment? What information will you share with your accountability team when you touch base with them this week?

DEVOTIONAL

My son, if you accept my words
and store up my commands within you,
² turning your ear to wisdom
and applying your heart to understanding—
³ indeed, if you call out for insight
and cry aloud for understanding,
⁴ and if you look for it as for silver
and search for it as for hidden treasure,
⁵ then you will understand the fear of the Lord
and find the knowledge of God.
⁶ For the Lord gives wisdom;
from his mouth come knowledge and understanding.
⁷ He holds success in store for the upright,
he is a shield to those whose walk is blameless,
⁸ for he guards the course of the just
and protects the way of his faithful ones.

PROVERBS 2:1-8

 Read Proverbs 2.

SWORD DRILL

Scripture - Which verse or group of verses stood out to you in the Proverbs reading? Write it/them below.

Wait - Take a few moments now to wait on the Holy Spirit. Put aside any thoughts and worries of the day. Meditate on the Scripture. Read the verse(s) above aloud, slowly and attentively. Then pause to let it sink in. Let the Holy Spirit speak to you.

Observe - What did you notice about the verse(s) from above? Was there something that the Holy Spirit spoke to you? Write your observation below.

Request - Ask God to show you where and how the Scripture and observation apply to your life. Write the application below.

Dedicate Yourself - Looking at how the Scripture applies to you, what is one thing that needs to change? Remember, this is not necessarily about something you need to do (or stop doing). Perhaps the change is in the way you see yourself or others.

FASTER SCALE

Adapted with permission from *The Genesis Process* by Michael Dye.

- • **Circle the behaviors that you identify with in each section.**
- • **Identify the most powerful behavior in each section and write it next to the corresponding heading.**
- • **Answer the following three questions:**
  1. How does it affect me? How do I feel in the moment?
  2. How does it affect the important people in my life?
  3. Why do I do this? What is the benefit for me?

RESTORATION _____

(Accepting life on God's terms, with trust, grace, mercy, vulnerability and gratitude.) No current secrets; working to resolve problems; identifying fears and feelings; keeping commitments to meetings, prayer, family, church, people, goals, and self; being open and honest, making eye contact; increasing in relationships with God and others; true accountability.

1. _____
2. _____
3. _____

FORGETTING PRIORITIES _____

(Start believing the present circumstances and moving away from trusting God. Denial; flight; a change in what's important; how you spend your time, energy, and thoughts.) Secrets; less time/energy for God, meetings, church; avoiding support and accountability people; superficial conversations; sarcasm; isolating; changes in goals; obsessed with relationships; breaking promises and commitments; neglecting family; preoccupation with material things, TV, computers, entertainment; procrastination; lying; overconfidence; bored; hiding money; image management; seeking to control situations and other people.

1. _____
   _____
2. _____
   _____
3. _____
   _____

ANXIETY

(A growing background noise of undefined fear; getting energy from emotions.) Worry, using profanity, being fearful; being resentful; replaying old, negative thoughts; perfectionism; judging other's motives; making goals and lists that you can't complete; mind reading; fantasy, codependent rescuing; sleep problems, trouble concentrating, seeking/creating drama; gossip; using over-the-counter medication for pain, sleep or weight control; flirting.

1. _____
   _____
2. _____
   _____
3. _____
   _____

SPEEDING UP

(Trying to outrun the anxiety which is usually the first sign of depression.) Super busy and always in a hurry (finding good reason to justify the work); workaholic; can't relax; avoiding slowing down; feeling driven; can't turn off thoughts; skipping meals; binge eating (usually at night); overspending; can't identify own feelings/needs; repetitive negative thoughts; irritable; dramatic mood swings; too much caffeine; over exercising; nervousness; difficulty being alone and/or with people; difficulty listening to others; making excuses for having to "do it all."

1. _____
   _____
2. _____
   _____
3. _____
   _____

TICKED OFF

(Getting adrenaline high on anger and aggression.) Procrastination causing crisis in money, work, and relationships; increased sarcasm; black and white (all or nothing) thinking; feeling alone; nobody understands; overreacting, road rage; constant resentments; pushing others away; increasing isolation; blaming; arguing; irrational thinking; can't take criticism; defensive; people avoiding you; needing to be right; digestive problems; headaches; obsessive (stuck) thoughts; can't forgive; feeling superior; using intimidation.

1. _____

2. _____

3. _____

EXHAUSTED _____

(Loss of physical and emotional energy; coming off the adrenaline high, and the onset of depression.) Depressed; panicked; confused; hopelessness; sleeping too much or too little; can't cope; overwhelmed; crying for "no reason"; can't think; forgetful; pessimistic; helpless; tired; numb; wanting to run; constant cravings for old coping behaviors; thinking of using sex, drugs, or alcohol; seeking old unhealthy people and places; really isolating; people angry with you; self abuse; suicidal thoughts; spontaneous crying; no goals; survival mode; not returning phone calls; missing work; irritability; no appetite.

1. _____

2. _____

3. _____

RELAPSE _____

(Returning to the place you swore you would never go again. Coping with life on your terms. You sitting in the driver's seat instead of God.) Giving up and giving in; out of control; lost in your addiction; lying to yourself and others; feeling you just can't manage without your coping behaviors, at least for now. The result is the reinforcement of shame, guilt and condemnation; and feelings of abandonment and being alone.

1. _____

2. _____

3. _____

GROUP CHECK-IN

COMPLETE 24 HOURS BEFORE GROUP

1 What is the lowest level you reached on the *FASTER Scale* this week?

2 What was the *Double Bind* you were dealing with?

3 Where are you on your *Commitment to Change* from our last meeting?

4 Have you lied to anyone this week either directly or indirectly?

5 What have you done to improve your relationship with your wife or other significant relationships this week?

PILLAR TWO
LESSON TWO

SECRECY

WORKBOOK PAGE / 68

- [ ] Pillar Two: Lesson Two Video
- [ ] Workbook Assignment
- [ ] Commitment to Change
- [ ] Devotional
- [ ] FASTER Scale
- [ ] Group Check-in

COMMITMENT TO CHANGE

1   What area do you need to change or what challenge are you facing next week?

2   What will it cost you emotionally if you do change? What fear will you have to face?

3   What will it cost you if you don't change?

4   What is your plan to maintain your restoration regarding these changes?

5   Who will you be accountable to as you pursue this commitment?

6   What are the details of this commitment? What information will you share with your accountability team when you touch base with them this week?

DEVOTIONAL

The Lord detests dishonest scales,
but accurate weights find favor with him.

² When pride comes, then comes disgrace,
but with humility comes wisdom.

³ The integrity of the upright guides them,
but the unfaithful are destroyed by their duplicity.

⁴ Wealth is worthless in the day of wrath,
but righteousness delivers from death.

⁵ The righteousness of the blameless makes their paths straight,
but the wicked are brought down by their own wickedness.

⁶ The righteousness of the upright delivers them,
but the unfaithful are trapped by evil desires.

⁷ Hopes placed in mortals die with them;
all the promise of their power comes to nothing.

⁸ The righteous person is rescued from trouble,
and it falls on the wicked instead.

PROVERBS 11:1-8

 Read Proverbs 11.

SWORD DRILL

Scripture - Which verse or group of verses stood out to you in the Proverbs reading? Write it/them below.

Wait - Take a few moments now to wait on the Holy Spirit. Put aside any thoughts and worries of the day. Meditate on the Scripture. Read the verse(s) above aloud, slowly and attentively. Then pause to let it sink in. Let the Holy Spirit speak to you.

Observe - What did you notice about the verse(s) from above? Was there something that the Holy Spirit spoke to you? Write your observation below.

Request - Ask God to show you where and how the Scripture and observation apply to your life. Write the application below.

Dedicate Yourself - Looking at how the Scripture applies to you, what is one thing that needs to change? Remember, this is not necessarily about something you need to do (or stop doing). Perhaps the change is in the way you see yourself or others.

FASTER SCALE

Adapted with permission from *The Genesis Process* by Michael Dye.

- **Circle the behaviors that you identify with in each section.**
- **Identify the most powerful behavior in each section and write it next to the corresponding heading.**
- **Answer the following three questions:**
  1. How does it affect me? How do I feel in the moment?
  2. How does it affect the important people in my life?
  3. Why do I do this? What is the benefit for me?

RESTORATION _____

(Accepting life on God's terms, with trust, grace, mercy, vulnerability and gratitude.)
No current secrets; working to resolve problems; identifying fears and feelings; keeping commitments to meetings, prayer, family, church, people, goals, and self; being open and honest, making eye contact; increasing in relationships with God and others; true accountability.

1. _____
2. _____
3. _____

FORGETTING PRIORITIES _____

(Start believing the present circumstances and moving away from trusting God. Denial; flight; a change in what's important; how you spend your time, energy, and thoughts.)
Secrets; less time/energy for God, meetings, church; avoiding support and accountability people; superficial conversations; sarcasm; isolating; changes in goals; obsessed with relationships; breaking promises and commitments; neglecting family; preoccupation with material things, TV, computers, entertainment; procrastination; lying; overconfidence; bored; hiding money; image management; seeking to control situations and other people.

1. _____
   _____
2. _____
   _____
3. _____
   _____

ANXIETY

(A growing background noise of undefined fear; getting energy from emotions.)
Worry, using profanity, being fearful; being resentful; replaying old, negative
thoughts; perfectionism; judging other's motives; making goals and lists that you
can't complete; mind reading; fantasy, codependent rescuing; sleep problems,
trouble concentrating, seeking/creating drama; gossip; using over-the-counter
medication for pain, sleep or weight control; flirting.

1. _____
   _____
2. _____
   _____
3. _____
   _____

SPEEDING UP

(Trying to outrun the anxiety which is usually the first sign of depression.) Super
busy and always in a hurry (finding good reason to justify the work); workaholic; can't
relax; avoiding slowing down; feeling driven; can't turn off thoughts; skipping meals;
binge eating (usually at night); overspending; can't identify own feelings/needs;
repetitive negative thoughts; irritable; dramatic mood swings; too much caffeine; over
exercising; nervousness; difficulty being alone and/or with people; difficulty listening
to others; making excuses for having to "do it all."

1. _____
   _____
2. _____
   _____
3. _____
   _____

TICKED OFF

(Getting adrenaline high on anger and aggression.) Procrastination causing crisis in
money, work, and relationships; increased sarcasm; black and white (all or nothing)
thinking; feeling alone; nobody understands; overreacting, road rage; constant resentments;
pushing others away; increasing isolation; blaming; arguing; irrational thinking; can't
take criticism; defensive; people avoiding you; needing to be right; digestive problems;
headaches; obsessive (stuck) thoughts; can't forgive; feeling superior; using intimidation.

1. _____
_____

2. _____
_____

3. _____
_____

EXHAUSTED _____

(Loss of physical and emotional energy; coming off the adrenaline high, and the onset of depression.) Depressed; panicked; confused; hopelessness; sleeping too much or too little; can't cope; overwhelmed; crying for "no reason"; can't think; forgetful; pessimistic; helpless; tired; numb; wanting to run; constant cravings for old coping behaviors; thinking of using sex, drugs, or alcohol; seeking old unhealthy people and places; really isolating; people angry with you; self abuse; suicidal thoughts; spontaneous crying; no goals; survival mode; not returning phone calls; missing work; irritability; no appetite.

1. _____
_____

2. _____
_____

3. _____
_____

RELAPSE _____

(Returning to the place you swore you would never go again. Coping with life on your terms. You sitting in the driver's seat instead of God.) Giving up and giving in; out of control; lost in your addiction; lying to yourself and others; feeling you just can't manage without your coping behaviors, at least for now. The result is the reinforcement of shame, guilt and condemnation; and feelings of abandonment and being alone.

1. _____
_____

2. _____
_____

3. _____
_____

GROUP CHECK-IN

COMPLETE 24 HOURS BEFORE GROUP

1   What is the lowest level you reached on the *FASTER Scale* this week?

2   What was the *Double Bind* you were dealing with?

3   Where are you on your *Commitment to Change* from our last meeting?

4   Have you lied to anyone this week either directly or indirectly?

5   What have you done to improve your relationship with your wife or other significant relationships this week?

PILLAR TWO
LESSON THREE

ISOLATION
WORKBOOK PAGE / 71

☐ Pillar Two: Lesson Three Video

☐ Workbook Assignment

☐ *Pure Desire* Reading

☐ Commitment to Change

☐ Devotional

☐ FASTER Scale

☐ Group Check-in

+   **Read Chapter 6 in *Pure Desire*. What were your observations?**

COMMITMENT TO CHANGE

1 What area do you need to change or what challenge are you facing next week?

2 What will it cost you emotionally if you do change? What fear will you have to face?

3 What will it cost you if you don't change?

4 What is your plan to maintain your restoration regarding these changes?

5 Who will you be accountable to as you pursue this commitment?

6 What are the details of this commitment? What information will you share with your accountability team when you touch base with them this week?

DEVOTIONAL

*⁹ How long will you lie there, you sluggard?
When will you get up from your sleep?
¹⁰ A little sleep, a little slumber,
a little folding of the hands to rest—
¹¹ and poverty will come on you like a thief
and scarcity like an armed man.*

*¹² A troublemaker and a villain,
who goes about with a corrupt mouth,
¹³ who winks maliciously with his eye,
signals with his feet
and motions with his fingers,
¹⁴ who plots evil with deceit in his heart—
he always stirs up conflict.
¹⁵ Therefore disaster will overtake him in an instant;
he will suddenly be destroyed—without remedy.*

PROVERBS 6:9-15

 Read Proverbs 6.

SWORD DRILL

S **cripture** - Which verse or group of verses stood out to you in the Proverbs reading? Write it/them below.

W **ait** - Take a few moments now to wait on the Holy Spirit. Put aside any thoughts and worries of the day. Meditate on the Scripture. Read the verse(s) above aloud, slowly and attentively. Then pause to let it sink in. Let the Holy Spirit speak to you.

O **bserve** - What did you notice about the verse(s) from above? Was there something that the Holy Spirit spoke to you? Write your observation below.

R **equest** - Ask God to show you where and how the Scripture and observation apply to your life. Write the application below.

D **edicate Yourself** - Looking at how the Scripture applies to you, what is one thing that needs to change? Remember, this is not necessarily about something you need to do (or stop doing). Perhaps the change is in the way you see yourself or others.

FASTER SCALE

Adapted with permission from *The Genesis Process* by Michael Dye.

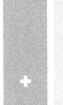

- **Circle the behaviors that you identify with in each section.**
- **Identify the most powerful behavior in each section and write it next to the corresponding heading.**
- **Answer the following three questions:**
  1. How does it affect me? How do I feel in the moment?
  2. How does it affect the important people in my life?
  3. Why do I do this? What is the benefit for me?

RESTORATION _____

(Accepting life on God's terms, with trust, grace, mercy, vulnerability and gratitude.)
No current secrets; working to resolve problems; identifying fears and feelings;
keeping commitments to meetings, prayer, family, church, people, goals, and self;
being open and honest, making eye contact; increasing in relationships with God and
others; true accountability.

1. _____
2. _____
3. _____

FORGETTING PRIORITIES _____

*(Start believing the present circumstances and moving away from trusting God. Denial;
flight; a change in what's important; how you spend your time, energy, and thoughts.)*
Secrets; less time/energy for God, meetings, church; avoiding support and accountability
people; superficial conversations; sarcasm; isolating; changes in goals; obsessed with
relationships; breaking promises and commitments; neglecting family; preoccupation
with material things, TV, computers, entertainment; procrastination; lying; overconfidence;
bored; hiding money; image management; seeking to control situations and other people.

1. _____
   _____
2. _____
   _____
3. _____
   _____

ANXIETY

(A growing background noise of undefined fear; getting energy from emotions.) Worry, using profanity, being fearful; being resentful; replaying old, negative thoughts; perfectionism; judging other's motives; making goals and lists that you can't complete; mind reading; fantasy, codependent rescuing; sleep problems, trouble concentrating, seeking/creating drama; gossip; using over-the-counter medication for pain, sleep or weight control; flirting.

1. _____
   _____

2. _____
   _____

3. _____
   _____

SPEEDING UP

(Trying to outrun the anxiety which is usually the first sign of depression.) Super busy and always in a hurry (finding good reason to justify the work); workaholic; can't relax; avoiding slowing down; feeling driven; can't turn off thoughts; skipping meals; binge eating (usually at night); overspending; can't identify own feelings/needs; repetitive negative thoughts; irritable; dramatic mood swings; too much caffeine; over exercising; nervousness; difficulty being alone and/or with people; difficulty listening to others; making excuses for having to "do it all."

1. _____
   _____

2. _____
   _____

3. _____
   _____

TICKED OFF

(Getting adrenaline high on anger and aggression.) Procrastination causing crisis in money, work, and relationships; increased sarcasm; black and white (all or nothing) thinking; feeling alone; nobody understands; overreacting, road rage; constant resentments; pushing others away; increasing isolation; blaming; arguing; irrational thinking; can't take criticism; defensive; people avoiding you; needing to be right; digestive problems; headaches; obsessive (stuck) thoughts; can't forgive; feeling superior; using intimidation.

1. _____

2. _____

3. _____

EXHAUSTED _____

(Loss of physical and emotional energy; coming off the adrenaline high, and the onset of depression.) Depressed; panicked; confused; hopelessness; sleeping too much or too little; can't cope; overwhelmed; crying for "no reason"; can't think; forgetful; pessimistic; helpless; tired; numb; wanting to run; constant cravings for old coping behaviors; thinking of using sex, drugs, or alcohol; seeking old unhealthy people and places; really isolating; people angry with you; self abuse; suicidal thoughts; spontaneous crying; no goals; survival mode; not returning phone calls; missing work; irritability; no appetite.

1. _____

2. _____

3. _____

RELAPSE _____

(Returning to the place you swore you would never go again. Coping with life on your terms. You sitting in the driver's seat instead of God.) Giving up and giving in; out of control; lost in your addiction; lying to yourself and others; feeling you just can't manage without your coping behaviors, at least for now. The result is the reinforcement of shame, guilt and condemnation; and feelings of abandonment and being alone.

1. _____

2. _____

3. _____

GROUP CHECK-IN

COMPLETE 24 HOURS BEFORE GROUP

1 What is the lowest level you reached on the *FASTER Scale* this week?

2 What was the *Double Bind* you were dealing with?

3 Where are you on your *Commitment to Change* from our last meeting?

4 Have you lied to anyone this week either directly or indirectly?

5 What have you done to improve your relationship with your wife or other significant relationships this week?

PILLAR TWO
LESSON FOUR

SHAME

WORKBOOK PAGE / 76

☐ Pillar Two: Lesson Four Video

☐ Workbook Assignment

☐ Commitment to Change

☐ Devotional

☐ FASTER Scale

☐ Group Check-in

COMMITMENT TO CHANGE

1   What area do you need to change or what challenge are you facing next week?

2   What will it cost you emotionally if you do change? What fear will you have to face?

3   What will it cost you if you don't change?

4   What is your plan to maintain your restoration regarding these changes?

5   Who will you be accountable to as you pursue this commitment?

6   What are the details of this commitment? What information will you share with your accountability team when you touch base with them this week?

DEVOTIONAL

Do not boast about tomorrow,
for you do not know what a day may bring.

² Let someone else praise you, and not your own mouth;
an outsider, and not your own lips.

³ Stone is heavy and sand a burden,
but a fool's provocation is heavier than both.

⁴ Anger is cruel and fury overwhelming,
but who can stand before jealousy?

⁵ Better is open rebuke
than hidden love.

⁶ Wounds from a friend can be trusted,
but an enemy multiplies kisses.

⁷ One who is full loathes honey from the comb,
but to the hungry even what is bitter tastes sweet.

⁸ Like a bird that flees its nest
is anyone who flees from home.

PROVERBS 27:1-8

 Read Proverbs 27.

SWORD DRILL

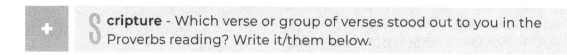

Scripture - Which verse or group of verses stood out to you in the Proverbs reading? Write it/them below.

Wait - Take a few moments now to wait on the Holy Spirit. Put aside any thoughts and worries of the day. Meditate on the Scripture. Read the verse(s) above aloud, slowly and attentively. Then pause to let it sink in. Let the Holy Spirit speak to you.

Observe - What did you notice about the verse(s) from above? Was there something that the Holy Spirit spoke to you? Write your observation below.

Request - Ask God to show you where and how the Scripture and observation apply to your life. Write the application below.

Dedicate Yourself - Looking at how the Scripture applies to you, what is one thing that needs to change? Remember, this is not necessarily about something you need to do (or stop doing). Perhaps the change is in the way you see yourself or others.

FASTER SCALE

Adapted with permission from *The Genesis Process* by Michael Dye.

- **Circle the behaviors that you identify with in each section.**
- **Identify the most powerful behavior in each section and write it next to the corresponding heading.**
- **Answer the following three questions:**
  1. How does it affect me? How do I feel in the moment?
  2. How does it affect the important people in my life?
  3. Why do I do this? What is the benefit for me?

RESTORATION _____

(Accepting life on God's terms, with trust, grace, mercy, vulnerability and gratitude.)
No current secrets; working to resolve problems; identifying fears and feelings; keeping commitments to meetings, prayer, family, church, people, goals, and self; being open and honest, making eye contact; increasing in relationships with God and others; true accountability.

1. _____
2. _____
3. _____

FORGETTING PRIORITIES _____

(Start believing the present circumstances and moving away from trusting God. Denial; flight; a change in what's important; how you spend your time, energy, and thoughts.)
Secrets; less time/energy for God, meetings, church; avoiding support and accountability people; superficial conversations; sarcasm; isolating; changes in goals; obsessed with relationships; breaking promises and commitments; neglecting family; preoccupation with material things, TV, computers, entertainment; procrastination; lying; overconfidence; bored; hiding money; image management; seeking to control situations and other people.

1. _____
   _____
2. _____
   _____
3. _____
   _____

ANXIETY

(A growing background noise of undefined fear; getting energy from emotions.)
Worry, using profanity, being fearful; being resentful; replaying old, negative thoughts; perfectionism; judging other's motives; making goals and lists that you can't complete; mind reading; fantasy, codependent rescuing; sleep problems, trouble concentrating, seeking/creating drama; gossip; using over-the-counter medication for pain, sleep or weight control; flirting.

1. _____

    _____

2. _____

    _____

3. _____

    _____

SPEEDING UP

(Trying to outrun the anxiety which is usually the first sign of depression.) Super busy and always in a hurry (finding good reason to justify the work); workaholic; can't relax; avoiding slowing down; feeling driven; can't turn off thoughts; skipping meals; binge eating (usually at night); overspending; can't identify own feelings/needs; repetitive negative thoughts; irritable; dramatic mood swings; too much caffeine; over exercising; nervousness; difficulty being alone and/or with people; difficulty listening to others; making excuses for having to "do it all."

1. _____

    _____

2. _____

    _____

3. _____

    _____

TICKED OFF

(Getting adrenaline high on anger and aggression.) Procrastination causing crisis in money, work, and relationships; increased sarcasm; black and white (all or nothing) thinking; feeling alone; nobody understands; overreacting, road rage; constant resentments; pushing others away; increasing isolation; blaming; arguing; irrational thinking; can't take criticism; defensive; people avoiding you; needing to be right; digestive problems; headaches; obsessive (stuck) thoughts; can't forgive; feeling superior; using intimidation.

1. _____

2. _____

3. _____

EXHAUSTED _____

(Loss of physical and emotional energy; coming off the adrenaline high, and the onset of depression.) Depressed; panicked; confused; hopelessness; sleeping too much or too little; can't cope; overwhelmed; crying for "no reason"; can't think; forgetful; pessimistic; helpless; tired; numb; wanting to run; constant cravings for old coping behaviors; thinking of using sex, drugs, or alcohol; seeking old unhealthy people and places; really isolating; people angry with you; self abuse; suicidal thoughts; spontaneous crying; no goals; survival mode; not returning phone calls; missing work; irritability; no appetite.

1. _____

2. _____

3. _____

RELAPSE _____

(Returning to the place you swore you would never go again. Coping with life on your terms. You sitting in the driver's seat instead of God.) Giving up and giving in; out of control; lost in your addiction; lying to yourself and others; feeling you just can't manage without your coping behaviors, at least for now. The result is the reinforcement of shame, guilt and condemnation; and feelings of abandonment and being alone.

1. _____

2. _____

3. _____

GROUP CHECK-IN

COMPLETE 24 HOURS BEFORE GROUP

1   What is the lowest level you reached on the *FASTER Scale* this week?

2   What was the *Double Bind* you were dealing with?

3   Where are you on your *Commitment to Change* from our last meeting?

4   Have you lied to anyone this week either directly or indirectly?

5   What have you done to improve your relationship with your wife or other significant relationships this week?

PILLAR TWO
LESSON FIVE

WARFARE
WORKBOOK PAGE / 83

☐ Pillar Two: Lesson Five Video

☐ Workbook Assignment

☐ *Pure Desire* Reading

☐ Commitment to Change

☐ Devotional

☐ FASTER Scale

☐ Group Check-in

+   **Read Chapter 7 in *Pure Desire*. What were your observations?**

COMMITMENT TO CHANGE

1   What area do you need to change or what challenge are you facing next week?

2   What will it cost you emotionally if you do change? What fear will you have to face?

3   What will it cost you if you don't change?

4   What is your plan to maintain your restoration regarding these changes?

5   Who will you be accountable to as you pursue this commitment?

6   What are the details of this commitment? What information will you share with your accountability team when you touch base with them this week?

DEVOTIONAL

The wicked flee though no one pursues,
but the righteous are as bold as a lion.

[2] When a country is rebellious, it has many rulers,
but a ruler with discernment and knowledge maintains order.

[3] A ruler who oppresses the poor
is like a driving rain that leaves no crops.

[4] Those who forsake instruction praise the wicked,
but those who heed it resist them.

[5] Evildoers do not understand what is right,
but those who seek the Lord understand it fully.

[6] Better the poor whose walk is blameless
than the rich whose ways are perverse.

[7] A discerning son heeds instruction,
but a companion of gluttons disgraces his father.

[8] Whoever increases wealth by taking interest or profit from the poor
amasses it for another, who will be kind to the poor.

PROVERBS 28:1-8

 Read Proverbs 28.

SWORD DRILL

Scripture - Which verse or group of verses stood out to you in the Proverbs reading? Write it/them below.

Wait - Take a few moments now to wait on the Holy Spirit. Put aside any thoughts and worries of the day. Meditate on the Scripture. Read the verse(s) above aloud, slowly and attentively. Then pause to let it sink in. Let the Holy Spirit speak to you.

Observe - What did you notice about the verse(s) from above? Was there something that the Holy Spirit spoke to you? Write your observation below.

Request - Ask God to show you where and how the Scripture and observation apply to your life. Write the application below.

Dedicate Yourself - Looking at how the Scripture applies to you, what is one thing that needs to change? Remember, this is not necessarily about something you need to do (or stop doing). Perhaps the change is in the way you see yourself or others.

FASTER SCALE

Adapted with permission from *The Genesis Process* by Michael Dye.

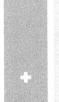

- + **Circle the behaviors that you identify with in each section.**
- + **Identify the most powerful behavior in each section and write it next to the corresponding heading.**
- + **Answer the following three questions:**
  1. How does it affect me? How do I feel in the moment?
  2. How does it affect the important people in my life?
  3. Why do I do this? What is the benefit for me?

RESTORATION _____

(Accepting life on God's terms, with trust, grace, mercy, vulnerability and gratitude.) No current secrets; working to resolve problems; identifying fears and feelings; keeping commitments to meetings, prayer, family, church, people, goals, and self; being open and honest, making eye contact; increasing in relationships with God and others; true accountability.

1. _____
2. _____
3. _____

FORGETTING PRIORITIES _____

(Start believing the present circumstances and moving away from trusting God. Denial; flight; a change in what's important; how you spend your time, energy, and thoughts.) Secrets; less time/energy for God, meetings, church; avoiding support and accountability people; superficial conversations; sarcasm; isolating; changes in goals; obsessed with relationships; breaking promises and commitments; neglecting family; preoccupation with material things, TV, computers, entertainment; procrastination; lying; overconfidence; bored; hiding money; image management; seeking to control situations and other people.

1. _____
   _____
2. _____
   _____
3. _____
   _____

ANXIETY

(A growing background noise of undefined fear; getting energy from emotions.) Worry, using profanity, being fearful; being resentful; replaying old, negative thoughts; perfectionism; judging other's motives; making goals and lists that you can't complete; mind reading; fantasy, codependent rescuing; sleep problems, trouble concentrating, seeking/creating drama; gossip; using over-the-counter medication for pain, sleep or weight control; flirting.

1. _____
   _____
2. _____
   _____
3. _____
   _____

SPEEDING UP

(Trying to outrun the anxiety which is usually the first sign of depression.) Super busy and always in a hurry (finding good reason to justify the work); workaholic; can't relax; avoiding slowing down; feeling driven; can't turn off thoughts; skipping meals; binge eating (usually at night); overspending; can't identify own feelings/needs; repetitive negative thoughts; irritable; dramatic mood swings; too much caffeine; over exercising; nervousness; difficulty being alone and/or with people; difficulty listening to others; making excuses for having to "do it all."

1. _____
   _____
2. _____
   _____
3. _____
   _____

TICKED OFF

(Getting adrenaline high on anger and aggression.) Procrastination causing crisis in money, work, and relationships; increased sarcasm; black and white (all or nothing) thinking; feeling alone; nobody understands; overreacting, road rage; constant resentments; pushing others away; increasing isolation; blaming; arguing; irrational thinking; can't take criticism; defensive; people avoiding you; needing to be right; digestive problems; headaches; obsessive (stuck) thoughts; can't forgive; feeling superior; using intimidation.

1. _____

_____

2. _____

_____

3. _____

_____

EXHAUSTED _____

(Loss of physical and emotional energy; coming off the adrenaline high, and the onset of depression.) Depressed; panicked; confused; hopelessness; sleeping too much or too little; can't cope; overwhelmed; crying for "no reason"; can't think; forgetful; pessimistic; helpless; tired; numb; wanting to run; constant cravings for old coping behaviors; thinking of using sex, drugs, or alcohol; seeking old unhealthy people and places; really isolating; people angry with you; self abuse; suicidal thoughts; spontaneous crying; no goals; survival mode; not returning phone calls; missing work; irritability; no appetite.

1. _____

_____

2. _____

_____

3. _____

_____

RELAPSE _____

(Returning to the place you swore you would never go again. Coping with life on your terms. You sitting in the driver's seat instead of God.) Giving up and giving in; out of control; lost in your addiction; lying to yourself and others; feeling you just can't manage without your coping behaviors, at least for now. The result is the reinforcement of shame, guilt and condemnation; and feelings of abandonment and being alone.

1. _____

_____

2. _____

_____

3. _____

_____

GROUP CHECK-IN

COMPLETE 24 HOURS BEFORE GROUP

1   What is the lowest level you reached on the *FASTER Scale* this week?

2   What was the *Double Bind* you were dealing with?

3   Where are you on your *Commitment to Change* from our last meeting?

4   Have you lied to anyone this week either directly or indirectly?

5   What have you done to improve your relationship with your wife or other significant relationships this week?

PILLAR THREE
LESSON ONE

LEARNING TO FACE THE PAIN
WORKBOOK PAGE / 92

☐ Pillar Three Intro Video

☐ Pillar Three: Lesson One Video

☐ Workbook Assignment

☐ *Pure Desire* Reading

☐ Commitment to Change

☐ Devotional

☐ FASTER Scale

☐ Group Check-in

+ **Read Chapter 8 in *Pure Desire*. What were your observations?**

COMMITMENT TO CHANGE

1 What area do you need to change or what challenge are you facing next week?

2 What will it cost you emotionally if you do change? What fear will you have to face?

3 What will it cost you if you don't change?

4 What is your plan to maintain your restoration regarding these changes?

5 Who will you be accountable to as you pursue this commitment?

6 What are the details of this commitment? What information will you share with your accountability team when you touch base with them this week?

DEVOTIONAL

² for gaining wisdom and instruction;
for understanding words of insight;
³ for receiving instruction in prudent behavior,
doing what is right and just and fair;
⁴ for giving prudence to those who are simple,
knowledge and discretion to the young—
⁵ let the wise listen and add to their learning,
and let the discerning get guidance—
⁶ for understanding proverbs and parables,
the sayings and riddles of the wise.

⁷ The fear of the Lord is the beginning of knowledge,
but fools despise wisdom and instruction.

PROVERBS 1:2-7

 Read Proverbs 1.

SWORD DRILL

S **cripture** - Which verse or group of verses stood out to you in the Proverbs reading? Write it/them below.

W **ait** - Take a few moments now to wait on the Holy Spirit. Put aside any thoughts and worries of the day. Meditate on the Scripture. Read the verse(s) above aloud, slowly and attentively. Then pause to let it sink in. Let the Holy Spirit speak to you.

O **bserve** - What did you notice about the verse(s) from above? Was there something that the Holy Spirit spoke to you? Write your observation below.

R **equest** - Ask God to show you where and how the Scripture and observation apply to your life. Write the application below.

D **edicate Yourself** - Looking at how the Scripture applies to you, what is one thing that needs to change? Remember, this is not necessarily about something you need to do (or stop doing). Perhaps the change is in the way you see yourself or others.

FASTER SCALE

Adapted with permission from *The Genesis Process* by Michael Dye.

- Circle the behaviors that you identify with in each section.
- Identify the most powerful behavior in each section and write it next to the corresponding heading.
- Answer the following three questions:
  1. How does it affect me? How do I feel in the moment?
  2. How does it affect the important people in my life?
  3. Why do I do this? What is the benefit for me?

RESTORATION _____

(Accepting life on God's terms, with trust, grace, mercy, vulnerability and gratitude.) No current secrets; working to resolve problems; identifying fears and feelings; keeping commitments to meetings, prayer, family, church, people, goals, and self; being open and honest, making eye contact; increasing in relationships with God and others; true accountability.

1. _____
2. _____
3. _____

FORGETTING PRIORITIES _____

(Start believing the present circumstances and moving away from trusting God. Denial; flight; a change in what's important; how you spend your time, energy, and thoughts.) Secrets; less time/energy for God, meetings, church; avoiding support and accountability people; superficial conversations; sarcasm; isolating; changes in goals; obsessed with relationships; breaking promises and commitments; neglecting family; preoccupation with material things, TV, computers, entertainment; procrastination; lying; overconfidence; bored; hiding money; image management; seeking to control situations and other people.

1. _____
   _____
2. _____
   _____
3. _____
   _____

ANXIETY

(A growing background noise of undefined fear; getting energy from emotions.) Worry, using profanity, being fearful; being resentful; replaying old, negative thoughts; perfectionism; judging other's motives; making goals and lists that you can't complete; mind reading; fantasy, codependent rescuing; sleep problems, trouble concentrating, seeking/creating drama; gossip; using over-the-counter medication for pain, sleep or weight control; flirting.

1. _____
_____
2. _____
_____
3. _____
_____

SPEEDING UP

(Trying to outrun the anxiety which is usually the first sign of depression.) Super busy and always in a hurry (finding good reason to justify the work); workaholic; can't relax; avoiding slowing down; feeling driven; can't turn off thoughts; skipping meals; binge eating (usually at night); overspending; can't identify own feelings/needs; repetitive negative thoughts; irritable; dramatic mood swings; too much caffeine; over exercising; nervousness; difficulty being alone and/or with people; difficulty listening to others; making excuses for having to "do it all."

1. _____
_____
2. _____
_____
3. _____
_____

TICKED OFF

(Getting adrenaline high on anger and aggression.) Procrastination causing crisis in money, work, and relationships; increased sarcasm; black and white (all or nothing) thinking; feeling alone; nobody understands; overreacting, road rage; constant resentments; pushing others away; increasing isolation; blaming; arguing; irrational thinking; can't take criticism; defensive; people avoiding you; needing to be right; digestive problems; headaches; obsessive (stuck) thoughts; can't forgive; feeling superior; using intimidation.

1. _____

_____

2. _____

_____

3. _____

_____

EXHAUSTED _____

(Loss of physical and emotional energy; coming off the adrenaline high, and the onset of depression.) Depressed; panicked; confused; hopelessness; sleeping too much or too little; can't cope; overwhelmed; crying for "no reason"; can't think; forgetful; pessimistic; helpless; tired; numb; wanting to run; constant cravings for old coping behaviors; thinking of using sex, drugs, or alcohol; seeking old unhealthy people and places; really isolating; people angry with you; self abuse; suicidal thoughts; spontaneous crying; no goals; survival mode; not returning phone calls; missing work; irritability; no appetite.

1. _____

_____

2. _____

_____

3. _____

_____

RELAPSE _____

(Returning to the place you swore you would never go again. Coping with life on your terms. You sitting in the driver's seat instead of God.) Giving up and giving in; out of control; lost in your addiction; lying to yourself and others; feeling you just can't manage without your coping behaviors, at least for now. The result is the reinforcement of shame, guilt and condemnation; and feelings of abandonment and being alone.

1. _____

_____

2. _____

_____

3. _____

_____

GROUP CHECK-IN

COMPLETE 24 HOURS BEFORE GROUP

1   What is the lowest level you reached on the *FASTER Scale* this week?

2   What was the *Double Bind* you were dealing with?

3   Where are you on your *Commitment to Change* from our last meeting?

4   Have you lied to anyone this week either directly or indirectly?

5   What have you done to improve your relationship with your wife or other significant relationships this week?

PILLAR THREE
LESSON TWO

BEING YOUR TRUE SELF
WORKBOOK PAGE / 100

- [ ] Pillar Three: Lesson Two Video
- [ ] Workbook Assignment
- [ ] Commitment to Change
- [ ] Devotional
- [ ] FASTER Scale
- [ ] Group Check-in

COMMITMENT TO CHANGE

1 What area do you need to change or what challenge are you facing next week?

2 What will it cost you emotionally if you do change? What fear will you have to face?

3 What will it cost you if you don't change?

4 What is your plan to maintain your restoration regarding these changes?

5 Who will you be accountable to as you pursue this commitment?

6 What are the details of this commitment? What information will you share with your accountability team when you touch base with them this week?

DEVOTIONAL

²¹ For your ways are in full view of the Lord,
and he examines all your paths.
²² The evil deeds of the wicked ensnare them;
the cords of their sins hold them fast.
²³ For lack of discipline they will die,
led astray by their own great folly.

PROVERBS 5:21-23

 Read Proverbs 5.

SWORD DRILL

S **cripture** - Which verse or group of verses stood out to you in the Proverbs reading? Write it/them below.

W **ait** - Take a few moments now to wait on the Holy Spirit. Put aside any thoughts and worries of the day. Meditate on the Scripture. Read the verse(s) above aloud, slowly and attentively. Then pause to let it sink in. Let the Holy Spirit speak to you.

O **bserve** - What did you notice about the verse(s) from above? Was there something that the Holy Spirit spoke to you? Write your observation below.

R **equest** - Ask God to show you where and how the Scripture and observation apply to your life. Write the application below.

D **edicate Yourself** - Looking at how the Scripture applies to you, what is one thing that needs to change? Remember, this is not necessarily about something you need to do (or stop doing). Perhaps the change is in the way you see yourself or others.

FASTER SCALE

Adapted with permission from *The Genesis Process* by Michael Dye.

- Circle the behaviors that you identify with in each section.
- Identify the most powerful behavior in each section and write it next to the corresponding heading.
- Answer the following three questions:
  1. How does it affect me? How do I feel in the moment?
  2. How does it affect the important people in my life?
  3. Why do I do this? What is the benefit for me?

RESTORATION _____

(Accepting life on God's terms, with trust, grace, mercy, vulnerability and gratitude.) No current secrets; working to resolve problems; identifying fears and feelings; keeping commitments to meetings, prayer, family, church, people, goals, and self; being open and honest, making eye contact; increasing in relationships with God and others; true accountability.

1. _____
2. _____
3. _____

FORGETTING PRIORITIES _____

(Start believing the present circumstances and moving away from trusting God. Denial; flight; a change in what's important; how you spend your time, energy, and thoughts.) Secrets; less time/energy for God, meetings, church; avoiding support and accountability people; superficial conversations; sarcasm; isolating; changes in goals; obsessed with relationships; breaking promises and commitments; neglecting family; preoccupation with material things, TV, computers, entertainment; procrastination; lying; overconfidence; bored; hiding money; image management; seeking to control situations and other people.

1. _____
   _____
2. _____
   _____
3. _____
   _____

ANXIETY

(A growing background noise of undefined fear; getting energy from emotions.)
Worry, using profanity, being fearful; being resentful; replaying old, negative
thoughts; perfectionism; judging other's motives; making goals and lists that you
can't complete; mind reading; fantasy, codependent rescuing; sleep problems,
trouble concentrating, seeking/creating drama; gossip; using over-the-counter
medication for pain, sleep or weight control; flirting.

1. _____

   _____

2. _____

   _____

3. _____

   _____

SPEEDING UP

(Trying to outrun the anxiety which is usually the first sign of depression.) Super
busy and always in a hurry (finding good reason to justify the work); workaholic; can't
relax; avoiding slowing down; feeling driven; can't turn off thoughts; skipping meals;
binge eating (usually at night); overspending; can't identify own feelings/needs;
repetitive negative thoughts; irritable; dramatic mood swings; too much caffeine; over
exercising; nervousness; difficulty being alone and/or with people; difficulty listening
to others; making excuses for having to "do it all."

1. _____

   _____

2. _____

   _____

3. _____

   _____

TICKED OFF

(Getting adrenaline high on anger and aggression.) Procrastination causing crisis in
money, work, and relationships; increased sarcasm; black and white (all or nothing)
thinking; feeling alone; nobody understands; overreacting, road rage; constant resentments;
pushing others away; increasing isolation; blaming; arguing; irrational thinking; can't
take criticism; defensive; people avoiding you; needing to be right; digestive problems;
headaches; obsessive (stuck) thoughts; can't forgive; feeling superior; using intimidation.

1. _____

_____

2. _____

_____

3. _____

_____

EXHAUSTED _____

(Loss of physical and emotional energy; coming off the adrenaline high, and the onset of depression.) Depressed; panicked; confused; hopelessness; sleeping too much or too little; can't cope; overwhelmed; crying for "no reason"; can't think; forgetful; pessimistic; helpless; tired; numb; wanting to run; constant cravings for old coping behaviors; thinking of using sex, drugs, or alcohol; seeking old unhealthy people and places; really isolating; people angry with you; self abuse; suicidal thoughts; spontaneous crying; no goals; survival mode; not returning phone calls; missing work; irritability; no appetite.

1. _____

_____

2. _____

_____

3. _____

_____

RELAPSE _____

(Returning to the place you swore you would never go again. Coping with life on your terms. You sitting in the driver's seat instead of God.) Giving up and giving in; out of control; lost in your addiction; lying to yourself and others; feeling you just can't manage without your coping behaviors, at least for now. The result is the reinforcement of shame, guilt and condemnation; and feelings of abandonment and being alone.

1. _____

_____

2. _____

_____

3. _____

_____

GROUP CHECK-IN

COMPLETE 24 HOURS BEFORE GROUP

1 What is the lowest level you reached on the *FASTER Scale* this week?

2 What was the *Double Bind* you were dealing with?

3 Where are you on your *Commitment to Change* from our last meeting?

4 Have you lied to anyone this week either directly or indirectly?

5 What have you done to improve your relationship with your wife or other significant relationships this week?

PILLAR THREE
LESSON THREE

LOVE, ACCEPTANCE, & FORGIVING
WORKBOOK PAGE / 106

☐ Pillar Three: Lesson Three Video

☐ Workbook Assignment

☐ Commitment to Change

☐ Devotional

☐ FASTER Scale

☐ Group Check-in

COMMITMENT TO CHANGE

1 What area do you need to change or what challenge are you facing next week?

2 What will it cost you emotionally if you do change? What fear will you have to face?

3 What will it cost you if you don't change?

4 What is your plan to maintain your restoration regarding these changes?

5 Who will you be accountable to as you pursue this commitment?

6 What are the details of this commitment? What information will you share with your accountability team when you touch base with them this week?

DEVOTIONAL

¹⁶ Better a little with the fear of the Lord
than great wealth with turmoil.

¹⁷ Better a small serving of vegetables with love
than a fattened calf with hatred.

¹⁸ A hot-tempered person stirs up conflict,
but the one who is patient calms a quarrel.

¹⁹ The way of the sluggard is blocked with thorns,
but the path of the upright is a highway.

²⁰ A wise son brings joy to his father,
but a foolish man despises his mother.

²¹ Folly brings joy to one who has no sense,
but whoever has understanding keeps a straight course.

²² Plans fail for lack of counsel,
but with many advisers they succeed.

²³ A person finds joy in giving an apt reply—
and how good is a timely word!

PROVERBS 15:16-23

 Read Proverbs 15.

SWORD DRILL

S cripture - Which verse or group of verses stood out to you in the Proverbs reading? Write it/them below.

W ait - Take a few moments now to wait on the Holy Spirit. Put aside any thoughts and worries of the day. Meditate on the Scripture. Read the verse(s) above aloud, slowly and attentively. Then pause to let it sink in. Let the Holy Spirit speak to you.

O bserve - What did you notice about the verse(s) from above? Was there something that the Holy Spirit spoke to you? Write your observation below.

R equest - Ask God to show you where and how the Scripture and observation apply to your life. Write the application below.

D edicate Yourself - Looking at how the Scripture applies to you, what is one thing that needs to change? Remember, this is not necessarily about something you need to do (or stop doing). Perhaps the change is in the way you see yourself or others.

FASTER SCALE

Adapted with permission from *The Genesis Process* by Michael Dye.

- **Circle the behaviors that you identify with in each section.**
- **Identify the most powerful behavior in each section and write it next to the corresponding heading.**
- **Answer the following three questions:**
  1. How does it affect me? How do I feel in the moment?
  2. How does it affect the important people in my life?
  3. Why do I do this? What is the benefit for me?

RESTORATION _____

(Accepting life on God's terms, with trust, grace, mercy, vulnerability and gratitude.) No current secrets; working to resolve problems; identifying fears and feelings; keeping commitments to meetings, prayer, family, church, people, goals, and self; being open and honest, making eye contact; increasing in relationships with God and others; true accountability.

1. _____
2. _____
3. _____

FORGETTING PRIORITIES _____

(Start believing the present circumstances and moving away from trusting God. Denial; flight; a change in what's important; how you spend your time, energy, and thoughts.) Secrets; less time/energy for God, meetings, church; avoiding support and accountability people; superficial conversations; sarcasm; isolating; changes in goals; obsessed with relationships; breaking promises and commitments; neglecting family; preoccupation with material things, TV, computers, entertainment; procrastination; lying; overconfidence; bored; hiding money; image management; seeking to control situations and other people.

1. _____
_____
2. _____
_____
3. _____
_____

ANXIETY

(A growing background noise of undefined fear; getting energy from emotions.)
Worry, using profanity, being fearful; being resentful; replaying old, negative
thoughts; perfectionism; judging other's motives; making goals and lists that you
can't complete; mind reading; fantasy, codependent rescuing; sleep problems,
trouble concentrating, seeking/creating drama; gossip; using over-the-counter
medication for pain, sleep or weight control; flirting.

1. _____
   _____

2. _____
   _____

3. _____
   _____

SPEEDING UP

(Trying to outrun the anxiety which is usually the first sign of depression.) Super
busy and always in a hurry (finding good reason to justify the work); workaholic; can't
relax; avoiding slowing down; feeling driven; can't turn off thoughts; skipping meals;
binge eating (usually at night); overspending; can't identify own feelings/needs;
repetitive negative thoughts; irritable; dramatic mood swings; too much caffeine; over
exercising; nervousness; difficulty being alone and/or with people; difficulty listening
to others; making excuses for having to "do it all."

1. _____
   _____

2. _____
   _____

3. _____
   _____

TICKED OFF

(Getting adrenaline high on anger and aggression.) Procrastination causing crisis in
money, work, and relationships; increased sarcasm; black and white (all or nothing)
thinking; feeling alone; nobody understands; overreacting, road rage; constant resentments;
pushing others away; increasing isolation; blaming; arguing; irrational thinking; can't
take criticism; defensive; people avoiding you; needing to be right; digestive problems;
headaches; obsessive (stuck) thoughts; can't forgive; feeling superior; using intimidation.

1. _____

2. _____

3. _____

EXHAUSTED _____

(Loss of physical and emotional energy; coming off the adrenaline high, and the onset of depression.) Depressed; panicked; confused; hopelessness; sleeping too much or too little; can't cope; overwhelmed; crying for "no reason"; can't think; forgetful; pessimistic; helpless; tired; numb; wanting to run; constant cravings for old coping behaviors; thinking of using sex, drugs, or alcohol; seeking old unhealthy people and places; really isolating; people angry with you; self abuse; suicidal thoughts; spontaneous crying; no goals; survival mode; not returning phone calls; missing work; irritability; no appetite.

1. _____

2. _____

3. _____

RELAPSE _____

(Returning to the place you swore you would never go again. Coping with life on your terms. You sitting in the driver's seat instead of God.) Giving up and giving in; out of control; lost in your addiction; lying to yourself and others; feeling you just can't manage without your coping behaviors, at least for now. The result is the reinforcement of shame, guilt and condemnation; and feelings of abandonment and being alone.

1. _____

2. _____

3. _____

GROUP CHECK-IN

COMPLETE 24 HOURS BEFORE GROUP

1   What is the lowest level you reached on the *FASTER Scale* this week?

2   What was the *Double Bind* you were dealing with?

3   Where are you on your *Commitment to Change* from our last meeting?

4   Have you lied to anyone this week either directly or indirectly?

5   What have you done to improve your relationship with your wife or other significant relationships this week?

PILLAR THREE
LESSON FOUR

SELF-CARE

WORKBOOK PAGE / 112

- ☐ Pillar Three: Lesson Four Video
- ☐ Workbook Assignment
- ☐ *Pure Desire* Reading
- ☐ Commitment to Change
- ☐ Devotional
- ☐ FASTER Scale
- ☐ Group Check-in

+   **Read Chapter 9 in *Pure Desire*. What were your observations?**

COMMITMENT TO CHANGE

1 What area do you need to change or what challenge are you facing next week?

2 What will it cost you emotionally if you do change? What fear will you have to face?

3 What will it cost you if you don't change?

4 What is your plan to maintain your restoration regarding these changes?

5 Who will you be accountable to as you pursue this commitment?

6 What are the details of this commitment? What information will you share with your accountability team when you touch base with them this week?

DEVOTIONAL

¹³ *Whoever scorns instruction will pay for it,*
but whoever respects a command is rewarded.

¹⁴ *The teaching of the wise is a fountain of life,*
turning a person from the snares of death.

¹⁵ *Good judgment wins favor,*
but the way of the unfaithful leads to their destruction.

¹⁶ *All who are prudent act with knowledge,*
but fools expose their folly.

¹⁷ *A wicked messenger falls into trouble,*
but a trustworthy envoy brings healing.

¹⁸ *Whoever disregards discipline comes to poverty and shame,*
but whoever heeds correction is honored.

¹⁹ *A longing fulfilled is sweet to the soul,*
but fools detest turning from evil.

²⁰ *Walk with the wise and become wise,*
for a companion of fools suffers harm.

PROVERBS 13:13-20

 Read Proverbs 13.

SWORD DRILL

Scripture - Which verse or group of verses stood out to you in the Proverbs reading? Write it/them below.

Wait - Take a few moments now to wait on the Holy Spirit. Put aside any thoughts and worries of the day. Meditate on the Scripture. Read the verse(s) above aloud, slowly and attentively. Then pause to let it sink in. Let the Holy Spirit speak to you.

Observe - What did you notice about the verse(s) from above? Was there something that the Holy Spirit spoke to you? Write your observation below.

Request - Ask God to show you where and how the Scripture and observation apply to your life. Write the application below.

Dedicate Yourself - Looking at how the Scripture applies to you, what is one thing that needs to change? Remember, this is not necessarily about something you need to do (or stop doing). Perhaps the change is in the way you see yourself or others.

FASTER SCALE

Adapted with permission from *The Genesis Process* by Michael Dye.

- Circle the behaviors that you identify with in each section.
- Identify the most powerful behavior in each section and write it next to the corresponding heading.
- Answer the following three questions:
  1. How does it affect me? How do I feel in the moment?
  2. How does it affect the important people in my life?
  3. Why do I do this? What is the benefit for me?

RESTORATION _____

(Accepting life on God's terms, with trust, grace, mercy, vulnerability and gratitude.) No current secrets; working to resolve problems; identifying fears and feelings; keeping commitments to meetings, prayer, family, church, people, goals, and self; being open and honest, making eye contact; increasing in relationships with God and others; true accountability.

1. _____
2. _____
3. _____

FORGETTING PRIORITIES _____

(Start believing the present circumstances and moving away from trusting God. Denial; flight; a change in what's important; how you spend your time, energy, and thoughts.) Secrets; less time/energy for God, meetings, church; avoiding support and accountability people; superficial conversations; sarcasm; isolating; changes in goals; obsessed with relationships; breaking promises and commitments; neglecting family; preoccupation with material things, TV, computers, entertainment; procrastination; lying; overconfidence; bored; hiding money; image management; seeking to control situations and other people.

1. _____
   _____
2. _____
   _____
3. _____
   _____

ANXIETY

(A growing background noise of undefined fear; getting energy from emotions.)
Worry, using profanity, being fearful; being resentful; replaying old, negative
thoughts; perfectionism; judging other's motives; making goals and lists that you
can't complete; mind reading; fantasy, codependent rescuing; sleep problems,
trouble concentrating, seeking/creating drama; gossip; using over-the-counter
medication for pain, sleep or weight control; flirting.

1. _____
   _____
2. _____
   _____
3. _____
   _____

SPEEDING UP

(Trying to outrun the anxiety which is usually the first sign of depression.) Super
busy and always in a hurry (finding good reason to justify the work); workaholic; can't
relax; avoiding slowing down; feeling driven; can't turn off thoughts; skipping meals;
binge eating (usually at night); overspending; can't identify own feelings/needs;
repetitive negative thoughts; irritable; dramatic mood swings; too much caffeine; over
exercising; nervousness; difficulty being alone and/or with people; difficulty listening
to others; making excuses for having to "do it all."

1. _____
   _____
2. _____
   _____
3. _____
   _____

TICKED OFF

(Getting adrenaline high on anger and aggression.) Procrastination causing crisis in
money, work, and relationships; increased sarcasm; black and white (all or nothing)
thinking; feeling alone; nobody understands; overreacting, road rage; constant resentments;
pushing others away; increasing isolation; blaming; arguing; irrational thinking; can't
take criticism; defensive; people avoiding you; needing to be right; digestive problems;
headaches; obsessive (stuck) thoughts; can't forgive; feeling superior; using intimidation.

1. _____

_____

2. _____

_____

3. _____

_____

EXHAUSTED _____

(Loss of physical and emotional energy; coming off the adrenaline high, and the onset of depression.) Depressed; panicked; confused; hopelessness; sleeping too much or too little; can't cope; overwhelmed; crying for "no reason"; can't think; forgetful; pessimistic; helpless; tired; numb; wanting to run; constant cravings for old coping behaviors; thinking of using sex, drugs, or alcohol; seeking old unhealthy people and places; really isolating; people angry with you; self abuse; suicidal thoughts; spontaneous crying; no goals; survival mode; not returning phone calls; missing work; irritability; no appetite.

1. _____

_____

2. _____

_____

3. _____

_____

RELAPSE _____

(Returning to the place you swore you would never go again. Coping with life on your terms. You sitting in the driver's seat instead of God.) Giving up and giving in; out of control; lost in your addiction; lying to yourself and others; feeling you just can't manage without your coping behaviors, at least for now. The result is the reinforcement of shame, guilt and condemnation; and feelings of abandonment and being alone.

1. _____

_____

2. _____

_____

3. _____

_____

GROUP CHECK-IN

COMPLETE 24 HOURS BEFORE GROUP

1   What is the lowest level you reached on the *FASTER Scale* this week?

2   What was the *Double Bind* you were dealing with?

3   Where are you on your *Commitment to Change* from our last meeting?

4   Have you lied to anyone this week either directly or indirectly?

5   What have you done to improve your relationship with your wife or other significant relationships this week?

PILLAR FOUR
LESSON ONE

YOU NEED A DAMAGE CONTROL PLAN
WORKBOOK PAGE / 120

- ☐ Pillar Four Intro Video
- ☐ Pillar Four: Lesson One Video
- ☐ Workbook Assignment
- ☐ *Pure Desire* Reading
- ☐ Commitment to Change
- ☐ Devotional
- ☐ FASTER Scale
- ☐ Group Check-in

+   **Read Chapter 10 in *Pure Desire*. What were your observations?**

COMMITMENT TO CHANGE

1   What area do you need to change or what challenge are you facing next week?

2   What will it cost you emotionally if you do change? What fear will you have to face?

3   What will it cost you if you don't change?

4   What is your plan to maintain your restoration regarding these changes?

5   Who will you be accountable to as you pursue this commitment?

6   What are the details of this commitment? What information will you share with your accountability team when you touch base with them this week?

DEVOTIONAL

*2 All a person's ways seem pure to them,
but motives are weighed by the Lord.*

*3 Commit to the Lord whatever you do,
and he will establish your plans.*

*4 The Lord works out everything to its proper end—
even the wicked for a day of disaster.*

*5 The Lord detests all the proud of heart.
Be sure of this: They will not go unpunished.*

*6 Through love and faithfulness sin is atoned for;
through the fear of the Lord evil is avoided.*

*7 When the Lord takes pleasure in anyone's way,
he causes their enemies to make peace with them.*

*8 Better a little with righteousness
than much gain with injustice.*

*9 In their hearts humans plan their course,
but the Lord establishes their steps.*

PROVERBS 16:2-9

 Read Proverbs 16.

SWORD DRILL

S **cripture** - Which verse or group of verses stood out to you in the Proverbs reading? Write it/them below.

W **ait** - Take a few moments now to wait on the Holy Spirit. Put aside any thoughts and worries of the day. Meditate on the Scripture. Read the verse(s) above aloud, slowly and attentively. Then pause to let it sink in. Let the Holy Spirit speak to you.

O **bserve** - What did you notice about the verse(s) from above? Was there something that the Holy Spirit spoke to you? Write your observation below.

R **equest** - Ask God to show you where and how the Scripture and observation apply to your life. Write the application below.

D **edicate Yourself** - Looking at how the Scripture applies to you, what is one thing that needs to change? Remember, this is not necessarily about something you need to do (or stop doing). Perhaps the change is in the way you see yourself or others.

FASTER SCALE

Adapted with permission from *The Genesis Process* by Michael Dye.

- **Circle the behaviors that you identify with in each section.**
- **Identify the most powerful behavior in each section and write it next to the corresponding heading.**
- **Answer the following three questions:**
  1. How does it affect me? How do I feel in the moment?
  2. How does it affect the important people in my life?
  3. Why do I do this? What is the benefit for me?

RESTORATION _____

(Accepting life on God's terms, with trust, grace, mercy, vulnerability and gratitude.) No current secrets; working to resolve problems; identifying fears and feelings; keeping commitments to meetings, prayer, family, church, people, goals, and self; being open and honest, making eye contact; increasing in relationships with God and others; true accountability.

1. _____
2. _____
3. _____

FORGETTING PRIORITIES _____

(Start believing the present circumstances and moving away from trusting God. Denial; flight; a change in what's important; how you spend your time, energy, and thoughts.) Secrets; less time/energy for God, meetings, church; avoiding support and accountability people; superficial conversations; sarcasm; isolating; changes in goals; obsessed with relationships; breaking promises and commitments; neglecting family; preoccupation with material things, TV, computers, entertainment; procrastination; lying; overconfidence; bored; hiding money; image management; seeking to control situations and other people.

1. _____
   _____
2. _____
   _____
3. _____
   _____

ANXIETY

(A growing background noise of undefined fear; getting energy from emotions.)
Worry, using profanity, being fearful; being resentful; replaying old, negative
thoughts; perfectionism; judging other's motives; making goals and lists that you
can't complete; mind reading; fantasy, codependent rescuing; sleep problems,
trouble concentrating, seeking/creating drama; gossip; using over-the-counter
medication for pain, sleep or weight control; flirting.

1. _____
   _____

2. _____
   _____

3. _____
   _____

SPEEDING UP

(Trying to outrun the anxiety which is usually the first sign of depression.) Super
busy and always in a hurry (finding good reason to justify the work); workaholic; can't
relax; avoiding slowing down; feeling driven; can't turn off thoughts; skipping meals;
binge eating (usually at night); overspending; can't identify own feelings/needs;
repetitive negative thoughts; irritable; dramatic mood swings; too much caffeine; over
exercising; nervousness; difficulty being alone and/or with people; difficulty listening
to others; making excuses for having to "do it all."

1. _____
   _____

2. _____
   _____

3. _____
   _____

TICKED OFF

(Getting adrenaline high on anger and aggression.) Procrastination causing crisis in
money, work, and relationships; increased sarcasm; black and white (all or nothing)
thinking; feeling alone; nobody understands; overreacting, road rage; constant resentments;
pushing others away; increasing isolation; blaming; arguing; irrational thinking; can't
take criticism; defensive; people avoiding you; needing to be right; digestive problems;
headaches; obsessive (stuck) thoughts; can't forgive; feeling superior; using intimidation.

1. _____

2. _____

3. _____

EXHAUSTED _____

(Loss of physical and emotional energy; coming off the adrenaline high, and the onset of depression.) Depressed; panicked; confused; hopelessness; sleeping too much or too little; can't cope; overwhelmed; crying for "no reason"; can't think; forgetful; pessimistic; helpless; tired; numb; wanting to run; constant cravings for old coping behaviors; thinking of using sex, drugs, or alcohol; seeking old unhealthy people and places; really isolating; people angry with you; self abuse; suicidal thoughts; spontaneous crying; no goals; survival mode; not returning phone calls; missing work; irritability; no appetite.

1. _____

2. _____

3. _____

RELAPSE _____

(Returning to the place you swore you would never go again. Coping with life on your terms. You sitting in the driver's seat instead of God.) Giving up and giving in; out of control; lost in your addiction; lying to yourself and others; feeling you just can't manage without your coping behaviors, at least for now. The result is the reinforcement of shame, guilt and condemnation; and feelings of abandonment and being alone.

1. _____

2. _____

3. _____

GROUP CHECK-IN

COMPLETE 24 HOURS BEFORE GROUP

1 What is the lowest level you reached on the *FASTER Scale* this week?

2 What was the *Double Bind* you were dealing with?

3 Where are you on your *Commitment to Change* from our last meeting?

4 Have you lied to anyone this week either directly or indirectly?

5 What have you done to improve your relationship with your wife or other significant relationships this week?

PILLAR FOUR
LESSON TWO

THE MATRIX OF ADDICTION
WORKBOOK PAGE / 125

☐ Pillar Four: Lesson Two Video

☐ Workbook Assignment

☐ Commitment to Change

☐ Devotional

☐ FASTER Scale

☐ Group Check-in

COMMITMENT TO CHANGE

1   What area do you need to change or what challenge are you facing next week?

2   What will it cost you emotionally if you do change? What fear will you have to face?

3   What will it cost you if you don't change?

4   What is your plan to maintain your restoration regarding these changes?

5   Who will you be accountable to as you pursue this commitment?

6   What are the details of this commitment? What information will you share with your accountability team when you touch base with them this week?

DEVOTIONAL

*² All a person's ways seem pure to them,
but motives are weighed by the Lord.*

*³ Commit to the Lord whatever you do,
and he will establish your plans.*

*⁴ The Lord works out everything to its proper end—
even the wicked for a day of disaster.*

*⁵ The Lord detests all the proud of heart.
Be sure of this: They will not go unpunished.*

*⁶ Through love and faithfulness sin is atoned for;
through the fear of the Lord evil is avoided.*

*⁷ When the Lord takes pleasure in anyone's way,
he causes their enemies to make peace with them.*

*⁸ Better a little with righteousness
than much gain with injustice.*

*⁹ In their hearts humans plan their course,
but the Lord establishes their steps.*

PROVERBS 18:1-8

 Read Proverbs 18.

SWORD DRILL

Scripture - Which verse or group of verses stood out to you in the Proverbs reading? Write it/them below.

Wait - Take a few moments now to wait on the Holy Spirit. Put aside any thoughts and worries of the day. Meditate on the Scripture. Read the verse(s) above aloud, slowly and attentively. Then pause to let it sink in. Let the Holy Spirit speak to you.

Observe - What did you notice about the verse(s) from above? Was there something that the Holy Spirit spoke to you? Write your observation below.

Request - Ask God to show you where and how the Scripture and observation apply to your life. Write the application below.

Dedicate Yourself - Looking at how the Scripture applies to you, what is one thing that needs to change? Remember, this is not necessarily about something you need to do (or stop doing). Perhaps the change is in the way you see yourself or others.

FASTER SCALE

Adapted with permission from *The Genesis Process* by Michael Dye.

- Circle the behaviors that you identify with in each section.
- Identify the most powerful behavior in each section and write it next to the corresponding heading.
- Answer the following three questions:
  1. How does it affect me? How do I feel in the moment?
  2. How does it affect the important people in my life?
  3. Why do I do this? What is the benefit for me?

RESTORATION _____

(Accepting life on God's terms, with trust, grace, mercy, vulnerability and gratitude.)
No current secrets; working to resolve problems; identifying fears and feelings; keeping commitments to meetings, prayer, family, church, people, goals, and self; being open and honest, making eye contact; increasing in relationships with God and others; true accountability.

1. _____
2. _____
3. _____

FORGETTING PRIORITIES _____

(Start believing the present circumstances and moving away from trusting God. Denial; flight; a change in what's important; how you spend your time, energy, and thoughts.)
Secrets; less time/energy for God, meetings, church; avoiding support and accountability people; superficial conversations; sarcasm; isolating; changes in goals; obsessed with relationships; breaking promises and commitments; neglecting family; preoccupation with material things, TV, computers, entertainment; procrastination; lying; overconfidence; bored; hiding money; image management; seeking to control situations and other people.

1. _____
2. _____
3. _____

ANXIETY _____

(A growing background noise of undefined fear; getting energy from emotions.)
Worry, using profanity, being fearful; being resentful; replaying old, negative
thoughts; perfectionism; judging other's motives; making goals and lists that you
can't complete; mind reading; fantasy, codependent rescuing; sleep problems,
trouble concentrating, seeking/creating drama; gossip; using over-the-counter
medication for pain, sleep or weight control; flirting.

1. _____
   _____
2. _____
   _____
3. _____
   _____

SPEEDING UP _____

(Trying to outrun the anxiety which is usually the first sign of depression.) Super
busy and always in a hurry (finding good reason to justify the work); workaholic; can't
relax; avoiding slowing down; feeling driven; can't turn off thoughts; skipping meals;
binge eating (usually at night); overspending; can't identify own feelings/needs;
repetitive negative thoughts; irritable; dramatic mood swings; too much caffeine; over
exercising; nervousness; difficulty being alone and/or with people; difficulty listening
to others; making excuses for having to "do it all."

1. _____
   _____
2. _____
   _____
3. _____
   _____

TICKED OFF _____

(Getting adrenaline high on anger and aggression.) Procrastination causing crisis in
money, work, and relationships; increased sarcasm; black and white (all or nothing)
thinking; feeling alone; nobody understands; overreacting, road rage; constant resentments;
pushing others away; increasing isolation; blaming; arguing; irrational thinking; can't
take criticism; defensive; people avoiding you; needing to be right; digestive problems;
headaches; obsessive (stuck) thoughts; can't forgive; feeling superior; using intimidation.

1. _____

2. _____

3. _____

EXHAUSTED _____

(Loss of physical and emotional energy; coming off the adrenaline high, and the onset of depression.) Depressed; panicked; confused; hopelessness; sleeping too much or too little; can't cope; overwhelmed; crying for "no reason"; can't think; forgetful; pessimistic; helpless; tired; numb; wanting to run; constant cravings for old coping behaviors; thinking of using sex, drugs, or alcohol; seeking old unhealthy people and places; really isolating; people angry with you; self abuse; suicidal thoughts; spontaneous crying; no goals; survival mode; not returning phone calls; missing work; irritability; no appetite.

1. _____

2. _____

3. _____

RELAPSE _____

(Returning to the place you swore you would never go again. Coping with life on your terms. You sitting in the driver's seat instead of God.) Giving up and giving in; out of control; lost in your addiction; lying to yourself and others; feeling you just can't manage without your coping behaviors, at least for now. The result is the reinforcement of shame, guilt and condemnation; and feelings of abandonment and being alone.

1. _____

2. _____

3. _____

GROUP CHECK-IN

COMPLETE 24 HOURS BEFORE GROUP

1   What is the lowest level you reached on the *FASTER Scale* this week?

2   What was the *Double Bind* you were dealing with?

3   Where are you on your *Commitment to Change* from our last meeting?

4   Have you lied to anyone this week either directly or indirectly?

5   What have you done to improve your relationship with your wife or other significant relationships this week?

PILLAR FOUR
LESSON THREE

WORKBOOK PAGE / 131

- [ ] Pillar Four: Lesson Three Video
- [ ] Workbook Assignment
- [ ] Commitment to Change
- [ ] Devotional
- [ ] FASTER Scale
- [ ] Group Check-in

COMMITMENT TO CHANGE

1   What area do you need to change or what challenge are you facing next week?

2   What will it cost you emotionally if you do change? What fear will you have to face?

3   What will it cost you if you don't change?

4   What is your plan to maintain your restoration regarding these changes?

5   Who will you be accountable to as you pursue this commitment?

6   What are the details of this commitment? What information will you share with your accountability team when you touch base with them this week?

DEVOTIONAL

¹⁶ Whoever keeps commandments keeps their life,
but whoever shows contempt for their ways will die.

¹⁷ Whoever is kind to the poor lends to the Lord,
and he will reward them for what they have done.

¹⁸ Discipline your children, for in that there is hope;
do not be a willing party to their death.

¹⁹ A hot-tempered person must pay the penalty;
rescue them, and you will have to do it again.

²⁰ Listen to advice and accept discipline,
and at the end you will be counted among the wise.

²¹ Many are the plans in a person's heart,
but it is the Lord's purpose that prevails.

²² What a person desires is unfailing love;
better to be poor than a liar.

²³ The fear of the Lord leads to life;
then one rests content, untouched by trouble.

PROVERBS 19:16-23

 Read Proverbs 19.

SWORD DRILL

S cripture - Which verse or group of verses stood out to you in the Proverbs reading? Write it/them below.

W ait - Take a few moments now to wait on the Holy Spirit. Put aside any thoughts and worries of the day. Meditate on the Scripture. Read the verse(s) above aloud, slowly and attentively. Then pause to let it sink in. Let the Holy Spirit speak to you.

O bserve - What did you notice about the verse(s) from above? Was there something that the Holy Spirit spoke to you? Write your observation below.

R equest - Ask God to show you where and how the Scripture and observation apply to your life. Write the application below.

D edicate Yourself - Looking at how the Scripture applies to you, what is one thing that needs to change? Remember, this is not necessarily about something you need to do (or stop doing). Perhaps the change is in the way you see yourself or others.

FASTER SCALE

Adapted with permission from *The Genesis Process* by Michael Dye.

- **Circle the behaviors that you identify with in each section.**
- **Identify the most powerful behavior in each section and write it next to the corresponding heading.**
- **Answer the following three questions:**
  1. How does it affect me? How do I feel in the moment?
  2. How does it affect the important people in my life?
  3. Why do I do this? What is the benefit for me?

RESTORATION _____

(Accepting life on God's terms, with trust, grace, mercy, vulnerability and gratitude.) No current secrets; working to resolve problems; identifying fears and feelings; keeping commitments to meetings, prayer, family, church, people, goals, and self; being open and honest, making eye contact; increasing in relationships with God and others; true accountability.

1. _____
2. _____
3. _____

FORGETTING PRIORITIES _____

(Start believing the present circumstances and moving away from trusting God. Denial; flight; a change in what's important; how you spend your time, energy, and thoughts.) Secrets; less time/energy for God, meetings, church; avoiding support and accountability people; superficial conversations; sarcasm; isolating; changes in goals; obsessed with relationships; breaking promises and commitments; neglecting family; preoccupation with material things, TV, computers, entertainment; procrastination; lying; overconfidence; bored; hiding money; image management; seeking to control situations and other people.

1. _____
   _____
2. _____
   _____
3. _____
   _____

ANXIETY

(A growing background noise of undefined fear; getting energy from emotions.)
Worry, using profanity, being fearful; being resentful; replaying old, negative
thoughts; perfectionism; judging other's motives; making goals and lists that you
can't complete; mind reading; fantasy, codependent rescuing; sleep problems,
trouble concentrating, seeking/creating drama; gossip; using over-the-counter
medication for pain, sleep or weight control; flirting.

1. _____
   _____
2. _____
   _____
3. _____
   _____

SPEEDING UP

(Trying to outrun the anxiety which is usually the first sign of depression.) Super
busy and always in a hurry (finding good reason to justify the work); workaholic; can't
relax; avoiding slowing down; feeling driven; can't turn off thoughts; skipping meals;
binge eating (usually at night); overspending; can't identify own feelings/needs;
repetitive negative thoughts; irritable; dramatic mood swings; too much caffeine; over
exercising; nervousness; difficulty being alone and/or with people; difficulty listening
to others; making excuses for having to "do it all."

1. _____
   _____
2. _____
   _____
3. _____
   _____

TICKED OFF

(Getting adrenaline high on anger and aggression.) Procrastination causing crisis in
money, work, and relationships; increased sarcasm; black and white (all or nothing)
thinking; feeling alone; nobody understands; overreacting, road rage; constant resentments;
pushing others away; increasing isolation; blaming; arguing; irrational thinking; can't
take criticism; defensive; people avoiding you; needing to be right; digestive problems;
headaches; obsessive (stuck) thoughts; can't forgive; feeling superior; using intimidation.

1. _____
   _____

2. _____
   _____

3. _____
   _____

EXHAUSTED _____

(Loss of physical and emotional energy; coming off the adrenaline high, and the onset of depression.) Depressed; panicked; confused; hopelessness; sleeping too much or too little; can't cope; overwhelmed; crying for "no reason"; can't think; forgetful; pessimistic; helpless; tired; numb; wanting to run; constant cravings for old coping behaviors; thinking of using sex, drugs, or alcohol; seeking old unhealthy people and places; really isolating; people angry with you; self abuse; suicidal thoughts; spontaneous crying; no goals; survival mode; not returning phone calls; missing work; irritability; no appetite.

1. _____
   _____

2. _____
   _____

3. _____
   _____

RELAPSE _____

(Returning to the place you swore you would never go again. Coping with life on your terms. You sitting in the driver's seat instead of God.) Giving up and giving in; out of control; lost in your addiction; lying to yourself and others; feeling you just can't manage without your coping behaviors, at least for now. The result is the reinforcement of shame, guilt and condemnation; and feelings of abandonment and being alone.

1. _____
   _____

2. _____
   _____

3. _____
   _____

GROUP CHECK-IN

COMPLETE 24 HOURS BEFORE GROUP

1 What is the lowest level you reached on the *FASTER Scale* this week?

2 What was the *Double Bind* you were dealing with?

3 Where are you on your *Commitment to Change* from our last meeting?

4 Have you lied to anyone this week either directly or indirectly?

5 What have you done to improve your relationship with your wife or other significant relationships this week?

PILLAR FOUR
LESSON FOUR

IDENTIFYING YOUR CRIPPLEDNESS
WORKBOOK PAGE / 139

- ☐ Pillar Four: Lesson Four Video
- ☐ Workbook Assignment
- ☐ *Pure Desire* Reading
- ☐ Commitment to Change
- ☐ Devotional
- ☐ FASTER Scale
- ☐ Group Check-in

+ **Read Chapter 11 in *Pure Desire*. What were your observations?**

COMMITMENT TO CHANGE

1 What area do you need to change or what challenge are you facing next week?

2 What will it cost you emotionally if you do change? What fear will you have to face?

3 What will it cost you if you don't change?

4 What is your plan to maintain your restoration regarding these changes?

5 Who will you be accountable to as you pursue this commitment?

6 What are the details of this commitment? What information will you share with your accountability team when you touch base with them this week?

DEVOTIONAL

⁷ The name of the righteous is used in blessings,
but the name of the wicked will rot.

⁸ The wise in heart accept commands,
but a chattering fool comes to ruin.

⁹ Whoever walks in integrity walks securely,
but whoever takes crooked paths will be found out.

¹⁰ Whoever winks maliciously causes grief,
and a chattering fool comes to ruin.

¹¹ The mouth of the righteous is a fountain of life,
but the mouth of the wicked conceals violence.

¹² Hatred stirs up conflict,
but love covers over all wrongs.

¹³ Wisdom is found on the lips of the discerning,
but a rod is for the back of one who has no sense.

¹⁴ The wise store up knowledge,
but the mouth of a fool invites ruin.

PROVERBS 10:7-14

 Read Proverbs 10.

SWORD DRILL

Scripture - Which verse or group of verses stood out to you in the Proverbs reading? Write it/them below.

Wait - Take a few moments now to wait on the Holy Spirit. Put aside any thoughts and worries of the day. Meditate on the Scripture. Read the verse(s) above aloud, slowly and attentively. Then pause to let it sink in. Let the Holy Spirit speak to you.

Observe - What did you notice about the verse(s) from above? Was there something that the Holy Spirit spoke to you? Write your observation below.

Request - Ask God to show you where and how the Scripture and observation apply to your life. Write the application below.

Dedicate Yourself - Looking at how the Scripture applies to you, what is one thing that needs to change? Remember, this is not necessarily about something you need to do (or stop doing). Perhaps the change is in the way you see yourself or others.

FASTER SCALE

Adapted with permission from *The Genesis Process* by Michael Dye.

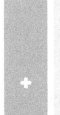

- Circle the behaviors that you identify with in each section.
- Identify the most powerful behavior in each section and write it next to the corresponding heading.
- Answer the following three questions:
  1. How does it affect me? How do I feel in the moment?
  2. How does it affect the important people in my life?
  3. Why do I do this? What is the benefit for me?

RESTORATION _____

(Accepting life on God's terms, with trust, grace, mercy, vulnerability and gratitude.) No current secrets; working to resolve problems; identifying fears and feelings; keeping commitments to meetings, prayer, family, church, people, goals, and self; being open and honest, making eye contact; increasing in relationships with God and others; true accountability.

1. _____
2. _____
3. _____

FORGETTING PRIORITIES _____

(Start believing the present circumstances and moving away from trusting God. Denial; flight; a change in what's important; how you spend your time, energy, and thoughts.) Secrets; less time/energy for God, meetings, church; avoiding support and accountability people; superficial conversations; sarcasm; isolating; changes in goals; obsessed with relationships; breaking promises and commitments; neglecting family; preoccupation with material things, TV, computers, entertainment; procrastination; lying; overconfidence; bored; hiding money; image management; seeking to control situations and other people.

1. _____
   _____
2. _____
   _____
3. _____
   _____

ANXIETY

(A growing background noise of undefined fear; getting energy from emotions.)
Worry, using profanity, being fearful; being resentful; replaying old, negative
thoughts; perfectionism; judging other's motives; making goals and lists that you
can't complete; mind reading; fantasy, codependent rescuing; sleep problems,
trouble concentrating, seeking/creating drama; gossip; using over-the-counter
medication for pain, sleep or weight control; flirting.

1. _____
   _____
2. _____
   _____
3. _____
   _____

SPEEDING UP

(Trying to outrun the anxiety which is usually the first sign of depression.) Super
busy and always in a hurry (finding good reason to justify the work); workaholic; can't
relax; avoiding slowing down; feeling driven; can't turn off thoughts; skipping meals;
binge eating (usually at night); overspending; can't identify own feelings/needs;
repetitive negative thoughts; irritable; dramatic mood swings; too much caffeine; over
exercising; nervousness; difficulty being alone and/or with people; difficulty listening
to others; making excuses for having to "do it all."

1. _____
   _____
2. _____
   _____
3. _____
   _____

TICKED OFF

(Getting adrenaline high on anger and aggression.) Procrastination causing crisis in
money, work, and relationships; increased sarcasm; black and white (all or nothing)
thinking; feeling alone; nobody understands; overreacting, road rage; constant resentments;
pushing others away; increasing isolation; blaming; arguing; irrational thinking; can't
take criticism; defensive; people avoiding you; needing to be right; digestive problems;
headaches; obsessive (stuck) thoughts; can't forgive; feeling superior; using intimidation.

1. _____
   _____
2. _____
   _____
3. _____
   _____

EXHAUSTED _____

(Loss of physical and emotional energy; coming off the adrenaline high, and the onset of depression.) Depressed; panicked; confused; hopelessness; sleeping too much or too little; can't cope; overwhelmed; crying for "no reason"; can't think; forgetful; pessimistic; helpless; tired; numb; wanting to run; constant cravings for old coping behaviors; thinking of using sex, drugs, or alcohol; seeking old unhealthy people and places; really isolating; people angry with you; self abuse; suicidal thoughts; spontaneous crying; no goals; survival mode; not returning phone calls; missing work; irritability; no appetite.

1. _____
   _____
2. _____
   _____
3. _____
   _____

RELAPSE _____

(Returning to the place you swore you would never go again. Coping with life on your terms. You sitting in the driver's seat instead of God.) Giving up and giving in; out of control; lost in your addiction; lying to yourself and others; feeling you just can't manage without your coping behaviors, at least for now. The result is the reinforcement of shame, guilt and condemnation; and feelings of abandonment and being alone.

1. _____
   _____
2. _____
   _____
3. _____
   _____

GROUP CHECK-IN

COMPLETE 24 HOURS BEFORE GROUP

1   What is the lowest level you reached on the *FASTER Scale* this week?

2   What was the *Double Bind* you were dealing with?

3   Where are you on your *Commitment to Change* from our last meeting?

4   Have you lied to anyone this week either directly or indirectly?

5   What have you done to improve your relationship with your wife or other significant relationships this week?

PILLAR FOUR
LESSON FIVE

GETTING UP OFF THE FLOOR
WORKBOOK PAGE / 147

- [ ] Pillar Four: Lesson Five Video
- [ ] Workbook Assignment
- [ ] Commitment to Change
- [ ] Devotional
- [ ] FASTER Scale
- [ ] Group Check-in

COMMITMENT TO CHANGE

1   What area do you need to change or what challenge are you facing next week?

2   What will it cost you emotionally if you do change? What fear will you have to face?

3   What will it cost you if you don't change?

4   What is your plan to maintain your restoration regarding these changes?

5   Who will you be accountable to as you pursue this commitment?

6   What are the details of this commitment? What information will you share with your accountability team when you touch base with them this week?

DEVOTIONAL

> *[5] Lord, you alone are my portion and my cup;*
> *you make my lot secure.*
>
> *[6] The boundary lines have fallen for me in pleasant places;*
> *surely I have a delightful inheritance.*
>
> *[7] I will praise the Lord, who counsels me;*
> *even at night my heart instructs me.*
>
> *[8] I keep my eyes always on the Lord.*
> *With him at my right hand, I will not be shaken.*
>
> PSALM 16:5-8

 Read Psalm 16.

SWORD DRILL

Scripture - Which verse or group of verses stood out to you in the Proverbs reading? Write it/them below.

Wait - Take a few moments now to wait on the Holy Spirit. Put aside any thoughts and worries of the day. Meditate on the Scripture. Read the verse(s) above aloud, slowly and attentively. Then pause to let it sink in. Let the Holy Spirit speak to you.

Observe - What did you notice about the verse(s) from above? Was there something that the Holy Spirit spoke to you? Write your observation below.

Request - Ask God to show you where and how the Scripture and observation apply to your life. Write the application below.

Dedicate Yourself - Looking at how the Scripture applies to you, what is one thing that needs to change? Remember, this is not necessarily about something you need to do (or stop doing). Perhaps the change is in the way you see yourself or others.

FASTER SCALE

Adapted with permission from *The Genesis Process* by Michael Dye.

- **Circle the behaviors that you identify with in each section.**
- **Identify the most powerful behavior in each section and write it next to the corresponding heading.**
- **Answer the following three questions:**
  1. How does it affect me? How do I feel in the moment?
  2. How does it affect the important people in my life?
  3. Why do I do this? What is the benefit for me?

RESTORATION _____

(Accepting life on God's terms, with trust, grace, mercy, vulnerability and gratitude.)
No current secrets; working to resolve problems; identifying fears and feelings; keeping commitments to meetings, prayer, family, church, people, goals, and self; being open and honest, making eye contact; increasing in relationships with God and others; true accountability.

1. _____
2. _____
3. _____

FORGETTING PRIORITIES _____

(Start believing the present circumstances and moving away from trusting God. Denial; flight; a change in what's important; how you spend your time, energy, and thoughts.)
Secrets; less time/energy for God, meetings, church; avoiding support and accountability people; superficial conversations; sarcasm; isolating; changes in goals; obsessed with relationships; breaking promises and commitments; neglecting family; preoccupation with material things, TV, computers, entertainment; procrastination; lying; overconfidence; bored; hiding money; image management; seeking to control situations and other people.

1. _____
_____
2. _____
_____
3. _____
_____

ANXIETY

(A growing background noise of undefined fear; getting energy from emotions.) Worry, using profanity, being fearful; being resentful; replaying old, negative thoughts; perfectionism; judging other's motives; making goals and lists that you can't complete; mind reading; fantasy, codependent rescuing; sleep problems, trouble concentrating, seeking/creating drama; gossip; using over-the-counter medication for pain, sleep or weight control; flirting.

1. _____
   _____
2. _____
   _____
3. _____
   _____

SPEEDING UP

(Trying to outrun the anxiety which is usually the first sign of depression.) Super busy and always in a hurry (finding good reason to justify the work); workaholic; can't relax; avoiding slowing down; feeling driven; can't turn off thoughts; skipping meals; binge eating (usually at night); overspending; can't identify own feelings/needs; repetitive negative thoughts; irritable; dramatic mood swings; too much caffeine; over exercising; nervousness; difficulty being alone and/or with people; difficulty listening to others; making excuses for having to "do it all."

1. _____
   _____
2. _____
   _____
3. _____
   _____

TICKED OFF

(Getting adrenaline high on anger and aggression.) Procrastination causing crisis in money, work, and relationships; increased sarcasm; black and white (all or nothing) thinking; feeling alone; nobody understands; overreacting, road rage; constant resentments; pushing others away; increasing isolation; blaming; arguing; irrational thinking; can't take criticism; defensive; people avoiding you; needing to be right; digestive problems; headaches; obsessive (stuck) thoughts; can't forgive; feeling superior; using intimidation.

1. _____

2. _____

3. _____

EXHAUSTED _____

(Loss of physical and emotional energy; coming off the adrenaline high, and the onset of depression.) Depressed; panicked; confused; hopelessness; sleeping too much or too little; can't cope; overwhelmed; crying for "no reason"; can't think; forgetful; pessimistic; helpless; tired; numb; wanting to run; constant cravings for old coping behaviors; thinking of using sex, drugs, or alcohol; seeking old unhealthy people and places; really isolating; people angry with you; self abuse; suicidal thoughts; spontaneous crying; no goals; survival mode; not returning phone calls; missing work; irritability; no appetite.

1. _____

2. _____

3. _____

RELAPSE _____

(Returning to the place you swore you would never go again. Coping with life on your terms. You sitting in the driver's seat instead of God.) Giving up and giving in; out of control; lost in your addiction; lying to yourself and others; feeling you just can't manage without your coping behaviors, at least for now. The result is the reinforcement of shame, guilt and condemnation; and feelings of abandonment and being alone.

1. _____

2. _____

3. _____

GROUP CHECK-IN

COMPLETE 24 HOURS BEFORE GROUP

1   What is the lowest level you reached on the *FASTER Scale* this week?

2   What was the *Double Bind* you were dealing with?

3   Where are you on your *Commitment to Change* from our last meeting?

4   Have you lied to anyone this week either directly or indirectly?

5   What have you done to improve your relationship with your wife or other significant relationships this week?

PILLAR FIVE
LESSON ONE

UNDERSTANDING FANTASIES
WORKBOOK PAGE / 158

☐ Pillar Five Intro Video

☐ Pillar Five: Lesson One Video

☐ Workbook Assignment

☐ *Pure Desire* Reading

☐ Commitment to Change

☐ Devotional

☐ FASTER Scale

☐ Group Check-in

+ **Read Chapter 12 in *Pure Desire*. What were your observations?**

COMMITMENT TO CHANGE

1 What area do you need to change or what challenge are you facing next week?

2 What will it cost you emotionally if you do change? What fear will you have to face?

3 What will it cost you if you don't change?

4 What is your plan to maintain your restoration regarding these changes?

5 Who will you be accountable to as you pursue this commitment?

6 What are the details of this commitment? What information will you share with your accountability team when you touch base with them this week?

DEVOTIONAL

A good name is more desirable than great riches;
to be esteemed is better than silver or gold.

² Rich and poor have this in common:
The Lord is the Maker of them all.

³ The prudent see danger and take refuge,
but the simple keep going and pay the penalty.

⁴ Humility is the fear of the Lord;
its wages are riches and honor and life.

⁵ In the paths of the wicked are snares and pitfalls,
but those who would preserve their life stay far from them.

⁶ Start children off on the way they should go,
and even when they are old they will not turn from it.

⁷ The rich rule over the poor,
and the borrower is slave to the lender.

⁸ Whoever sows injustice reaps calamity,
and the rod they wield in fury will be broken.

PROVERBS 22:1-8

 Read Proverbs 22.

SWORD DRILL

S **cripture** - Which verse or group of verses stood out to you in the Proverbs reading? Write it/them below.

W **ait** - Take a few moments now to wait on the Holy Spirit. Put aside any thoughts and worries of the day. Meditate on the Scripture. Read the verse(s) above aloud, slowly and attentively. Then pause to let it sink in. Let the Holy Spirit speak to you.

O **bserve** - What did you notice about the verse(s) from above? Was there something that the Holy Spirit spoke to you? Write your observation below.

R **equest** - Ask God to show you where and how the Scripture and observation apply to your life. Write the application below.

D **edicate Yourself** - Looking at how the Scripture applies to you, what is one thing that needs to change? Remember, this is not necessarily about something you need to do (or stop doing). Perhaps the change is in the way you see yourself or others.

FASTER SCALE

Adapted with permission from *The Genesis Process* by Michael Dye.

+ **Circle the behaviors that you identify with in each section.**

+ **Identify the most powerful behavior in each section and write it next to the corresponding heading.**

+ **Answer the following three questions:**

  1. How does it affect me? How do I feel in the moment?

  2. How does it affect the important people in my life?

  3. Why do I do this? What is the benefit for me?

RESTORATION _____

(Accepting life on God's terms, with trust, grace, mercy, vulnerability and gratitude.) No current secrets; working to resolve problems; identifying fears and feelings; keeping commitments to meetings, prayer, family, church, people, goals, and self; being open and honest, making eye contact; increasing in relationships with God and others; true accountability.

1. _____

2. _____

3. _____

FORGETTING PRIORITIES _____

(Start believing the present circumstances and moving away from trusting God. Denial; flight; a change in what's important; how you spend your time, energy, and thoughts.) Secrets; less time/energy for God, meetings, church; avoiding support and accountability people; superficial conversations; sarcasm; isolating; changes in goals; obsessed with relationships; breaking promises and commitments; neglecting family; preoccupation with material things, TV, computers, entertainment; procrastination; lying; overconfidence; bored; hiding money; image management; seeking to control situations and other people.

1. _____
   _____

2. _____
   _____

3. _____
   _____

ANXIETY

(A growing background noise of undefined fear; getting energy from emotions.) Worry, using profanity, being fearful; being resentful; replaying old, negative thoughts; perfectionism; judging other's motives; making goals and lists that you can't complete; mind reading; fantasy, codependent rescuing; sleep problems, trouble concentrating, seeking/creating drama; gossip; using over-the-counter medication for pain, sleep or weight control; flirting.

1. _____
   _____

2. _____
   _____

3. _____
   _____

SPEEDING UP

(Trying to outrun the anxiety which is usually the first sign of depression.) Super busy and always in a hurry (finding good reason to justify the work); workaholic; can't relax; avoiding slowing down; feeling driven; can't turn off thoughts; skipping meals; binge eating (usually at night); overspending; can't identify own feelings/needs; repetitive negative thoughts; irritable; dramatic mood swings; too much caffeine; over exercising; nervousness; difficulty being alone and/or with people; difficulty listening to others; making excuses for having to "do it all."

1. _____
   _____

2. _____
   _____

3. _____
   _____

TICKED OFF

(Getting adrenaline high on anger and aggression.) Procrastination causing crisis in money, work, and relationships; increased sarcasm; black and white (all or nothing) thinking; feeling alone; nobody understands; overreacting, road rage; constant resentments; pushing others away; increasing isolation; blaming; arguing; irrational thinking; can't take criticism; defensive; people avoiding you; needing to be right; digestive problems; headaches; obsessive (stuck) thoughts; can't forgive; feeling superior; using intimidation.

1. _____
   _____

2. _____
   _____

3. _____
   _____

EXHAUSTED _____

(Loss of physical and emotional energy; coming off the adrenaline high, and the onset of depression.) Depressed; panicked; confused; hopelessness; sleeping too much or too little; can't cope; overwhelmed; crying for "no reason"; can't think; forgetful; pessimistic; helpless; tired; numb; wanting to run; constant cravings for old coping behaviors; thinking of using sex, drugs, or alcohol; seeking old unhealthy people and places; really isolating; people angry with you; self abuse; suicidal thoughts; spontaneous crying; no goals; survival mode; not returning phone calls; missing work; irritability; no appetite.

1. _____
   _____

2. _____
   _____

3. _____
   _____

RELAPSE _____

(Returning to the place you swore you would never go again. Coping with life on your terms. You sitting in the driver's seat instead of God.) Giving up and giving in; out of control; lost in your addiction; lying to yourself and others; feeling you just can't manage without your coping behaviors, at least for now. The result is the reinforcement of shame, guilt and condemnation; and feelings of abandonment and being alone.

1. _____
   _____

2. _____
   _____

3. _____
   _____

GROUP CHECK-IN

COMPLETE 24 HOURS BEFORE GROUP

1 What is the lowest level you reached on the *FASTER Scale* this week?

2 What was the *Double Bind* you were dealing with?

3 Where are you on your *Commitment to Change* from our last meeting?

4 Have you lied to anyone this week either directly or indirectly?

5 What have you done to improve your relationship with your wife or other significant relationships this week?

PILLAR FIVE
LESSON TWO

TRUSTING GOD IN THE MOMENT
WORKBOOK PAGES / 165

☐ Pillar Five: Lesson Two Video

☐ Workbook Assignment

☐ *Pure Desire* Reading

☐ Commitment to Change

☐ Devotional

☐ FASTER Scale

☐ Group Check-in

+   **Read Chapter 13 in *Pure Desire*. What were your observations?**

COMMITMENT TO CHANGE

1   What area do you need to change or what challenge are you facing next week?

2   What will it cost you emotionally if you do change? What fear will you have to face?

3   What will it cost you if you don't change?

4   What is your plan to maintain your restoration regarding these changes?

5   Who will you be accountable to as you pursue this commitment?

6   What are the details of this commitment? What information will you share with your accountability team when you touch base with them this week?

DEVOTIONAL

*Whoever remains stiff-necked after many rebukes
will suddenly be destroyed—without remedy.*

*2 When the righteous thrive, the people rejoice;
when the wicked rule, the people groan.*

*3 A man who loves wisdom brings joy to his father,
but a companion of prostitutes squanders his wealth.*

*4 By justice a king gives a country stability,
but those who are greedy for bribes tear it down.*

*5 Those who flatter their neighbors
are spreading nets for their feet.*

*6 Evildoers are snared by their own sin,
but the righteous shout for joy and are glad.*

*7 The righteous care about justice for the poor,
but the wicked have no such concern.*

*8 Mockers stir up a city,
but the wise turn away anger.*

PROVERBS 29:1-8

 Read Proverbs 29.

SWORD DRILL

S **cripture** - Which verse or group of verses stood out to you in the Proverbs reading? Write it/them below.

W **ait** - Take a few moments now to wait on the Holy Spirit. Put aside any thoughts and worries of the day. Meditate on the Scripture. Read the verse(s) above aloud, slowly and attentively. Then pause to let it sink in. Let the Holy Spirit speak to you.

O **bserve** - What did you notice about the verse(s) from above? Was there something that the Holy Spirit spoke to you? Write your observation below.

R **equest** - Ask God to show you where and how the Scripture and observation apply to your life. Write the application below.

D **edicate Yourself** - Looking at how the Scripture applies to you, what is one thing that needs to change? Remember, this is not necessarily about something you need to do (or stop doing). Perhaps the change is in the way you see yourself or others.

FASTER SCALE

Adapted with permission from *The Genesis Process* by Michael Dye.

- **Circle the behaviors that you identify with in each section.**
- **Identify the most powerful behavior in each section and write it next to the corresponding heading.**
- **Answer the following three questions:**
  1. How does it affect me? How do I feel in the moment?
  2. How does it affect the important people in my life?
  3. Why do I do this? What is the benefit for me?

RESTORATION _____

(Accepting life on God's terms, with trust, grace, mercy, vulnerability and gratitude.) No current secrets; working to resolve problems; identifying fears and feelings; keeping commitments to meetings, prayer, family, church, people, goals, and self; being open and honest, making eye contact; increasing in relationships with God and others; true accountability.

1. _____

2. _____

3. _____

FORGETTING PRIORITIES _____

(Start believing the present circumstances and moving away from trusting God. Denial; flight; a change in what's important; how you spend your time, energy, and thoughts.) Secrets; less time/energy for God, meetings, church; avoiding support and accountability people; superficial conversations; sarcasm; isolating; changes in goals; obsessed with relationships; breaking promises and commitments; neglecting family; preoccupation with material things, TV, computers, entertainment; procrastination; lying; overconfidence; bored; hiding money; image management; seeking to control situations and other people.

1. _____
   _____

2. _____
   _____

3. _____
   _____

ANXIETY

(A growing background noise of undefined fear; getting energy from emotions.) Worry, using profanity, being fearful; being resentful; replaying old, negative thoughts; perfectionism; judging other's motives; making goals and lists that you can't complete; mind reading; fantasy, codependent rescuing; sleep problems, trouble concentrating, seeking/creating drama; gossip; using over-the-counter medication for pain, sleep or weight control; flirting.

1. _____
   _____
2. _____
   _____
3. _____
   _____

SPEEDING UP

(Trying to outrun the anxiety which is usually the first sign of depression.) Super busy and always in a hurry (finding good reason to justify the work); workaholic; can't relax; avoiding slowing down; feeling driven; can't turn off thoughts; skipping meals; binge eating (usually at night); overspending; can't identify own feelings/needs; repetitive negative thoughts; irritable; dramatic mood swings; too much caffeine; over exercising; nervousness; difficulty being alone and/or with people; difficulty listening to others; making excuses for having to "do it all."

1. _____
   _____
2. _____
   _____
3. _____
   _____

TICKED OFF

(Getting adrenaline high on anger and aggression.) Procrastination causing crisis in money, work, and relationships; increased sarcasm; black and white (all or nothing) thinking; feeling alone; nobody understands; overreacting, road rage; constant resentments; pushing others away; increasing isolation; blaming; arguing; irrational thinking; can't take criticism; defensive; people avoiding you; needing to be right; digestive problems; headaches; obsessive (stuck) thoughts; can't forgive; feeling superior; using intimidation.

1. _____

2. _____

3. _____

EXHAUSTED _____

(Loss of physical and emotional energy; coming off the adrenaline high, and the onset of depression.) Depressed; panicked; confused; hopelessness; sleeping too much or too little; can't cope; overwhelmed; crying for "no reason"; can't think; forgetful; pessimistic; helpless; tired; numb; wanting to run; constant cravings for old coping behaviors; thinking of using sex, drugs, or alcohol; seeking old unhealthy people and places; really isolating; people angry with you; self abuse; suicidal thoughts; spontaneous crying; no goals; survival mode; not returning phone calls; missing work; irritability; no appetite.

1. _____

2. _____

3. _____

RELAPSE _____

(Returning to the place you swore you would never go again. Coping with life on your terms. You sitting in the driver's seat instead of God.) Giving up and giving in; out of control; lost in your addiction; lying to yourself and others; feeling you just can't manage without your coping behaviors, at least for now. The result is the reinforcement of shame, guilt and condemnation; and feelings of abandonment and being alone.

1. _____

2. _____

3. _____

GROUP CHECK-IN

COMPLETE 24 HOURS BEFORE GROUP

1   What is the lowest level you reached on the *FASTER Scale* this week?

2   What was the *Double Bind* you were dealing with?

3   Where are you on your *Commitment to Change* from our last meeting?

4   Have you lied to anyone this week either directly or indirectly?

5   What have you done to improve your relationship with your wife or other significant relationships this week?

PILLAR FIVE
LESSON THREE

TRAINING EXERCISES
WORKBOOK PAGE / 174

☐ Pillar Five: Lesson Three Video

☐ Workbook Assignment

☐ Commitment to Change

☐ Devotional

☐ FASTER Scale

☐ Group Check-in

COMMITMENT TO CHANGE

1 What area do you need to change or what challenge are you facing next week?

2 What will it cost you emotionally if you do change? What fear will you have to face?

3 What will it cost you if you don't change?

4 What is your plan to maintain your restoration regarding these changes?

5 Who will you be accountable to as you pursue this commitment?

6 What are the details of this commitment? What information will you share with your accountability team when you touch base with them this week?

DEVOTIONAL

Do not envy the wicked,
do not desire their company;
² for their hearts plot violence,
and their lips talk about making trouble.

³ By wisdom a house is built,
and through understanding it is established;
⁴ through knowledge its rooms are filled
with rare and beautiful treasures.

⁵ The wise prevail through great power,
and those who have knowledge muster their strength.
⁶ Surely you need guidance to wage war,
and victory is won through many advisers.

⁷ Wisdom is too high for fools;
in the assembly at the gate they must not open their mouths.

PROVERBS 24:1-7

 Read Proverbs 24.

SWORD DRILL

Scripture - Which verse or group of verses stood out to you in the Proverbs reading? Write it/them below.

Wait - Take a few moments now to wait on the Holy Spirit. Put aside any thoughts and worries of the day. Meditate on the Scripture. Read the verse(s) above aloud, slowly and attentively. Then pause to let it sink in. Let the Holy Spirit speak to you.

Observe - What did you notice about the verse(s) from above? Was there something that the Holy Spirit spoke to you? Write your observation below.

Request - Ask God to show you where and how the Scripture and observation apply to your life. Write the application below.

Dedicate Yourself - Looking at how the Scripture applies to you, what is one thing that needs to change? Remember, this is not necessarily about something you need to do (or stop doing). Perhaps the change is in the way you see yourself or others.

FASTER SCALE

Adapted with permission from *The Genesis Process* by Michael Dye.

- Circle the behaviors that you identify with in each section.
- Identify the most powerful behavior in each section and write it next to the corresponding heading.
- Answer the following three questions:
  1. How does it affect me? How do I feel in the moment?
  2. How does it affect the important people in my life?
  3. Why do I do this? What is the benefit for me?

RESTORATION _____

(Accepting life on God's terms, with trust, grace, mercy, vulnerability and gratitude.) No current secrets; working to resolve problems; identifying fears and feelings; keeping commitments to meetings, prayer, family, church, people, goals, and self; being open and honest, making eye contact; increasing in relationships with God and others; true accountability.

1. _____
2. _____
3. _____

FORGETTING PRIORITIES _____

(Start believing the present circumstances and moving away from trusting God. Denial; flight; a change in what's important; how you spend your time, energy, and thoughts.) Secrets; less time/energy for God, meetings, church; avoiding support and accountability people; superficial conversations; sarcasm; isolating; changes in goals; obsessed with relationships; breaking promises and commitments; neglecting family; preoccupation with material things, TV, computers, entertainment; procrastination; lying; overconfidence; bored; hiding money; image management; seeking to control situations and other people.

1. _____
   _____
2. _____
   _____
3. _____
   _____

ANXIETY

(A growing background noise of undefined fear; getting energy from emotions.)
Worry, using profanity, being fearful; being resentful; replaying old, negative
thoughts; perfectionism; judging other's motives; making goals and lists that you
can't complete; mind reading; fantasy, codependent rescuing; sleep problems,
trouble concentrating, seeking/creating drama; gossip; using over-the-counter
medication for pain, sleep or weight control; flirting.

1. _____

   _____

2. _____

   _____

3. _____

   _____

SPEEDING UP

(Trying to outrun the anxiety which is usually the first sign of depression.) Super
busy and always in a hurry (finding good reason to justify the work); workaholic; can't
relax; avoiding slowing down; feeling driven; can't turn off thoughts; skipping meals;
binge eating (usually at night); overspending; can't identify own feelings/needs;
repetitive negative thoughts; irritable; dramatic mood swings; too much caffeine; over
exercising; nervousness; difficulty being alone and/or with people; difficulty listening
to others; making excuses for having to "do it all."

1. _____

   _____

2. _____

   _____

3. _____

   _____

TICKED OFF

(Getting adrenaline high on anger and aggression.) Procrastination causing crisis in
money, work, and relationships; increased sarcasm; black and white (all or nothing)
thinking; feeling alone; nobody understands; overreacting, road rage; constant resentments;
pushing others away; increasing isolation; blaming; arguing; irrational thinking; can't
take criticism; defensive; people avoiding you; needing to be right; digestive problems;
headaches; obsessive (stuck) thoughts; can't forgive; feeling superior; using intimidation.

1. _____
   _____
2. _____
   _____
3. _____
   _____

EXHAUSTED _____

(Loss of physical and emotional energy; coming off the adrenaline high, and the onset of depression.) Depressed; panicked; confused; hopelessness; sleeping too much or too little; can't cope; overwhelmed; crying for "no reason"; can't think; forgetful; pessimistic; helpless; tired; numb; wanting to run; constant cravings for old coping behaviors; thinking of using sex, drugs, or alcohol; seeking old unhealthy people and places; really isolating; people angry with you; self abuse; suicidal thoughts; spontaneous crying; no goals; survival mode; not returning phone calls; missing work; irritability; no appetite.

1. _____
   _____
2. _____
   _____
3. _____
   _____

RELAPSE _____

(Returning to the place you swore you would never go again. Coping with life on your terms. You sitting in the driver's seat instead of God.) Giving up and giving in; out of control; lost in your addiction; lying to yourself and others; feeling you just can't manage without your coping behaviors, at least for now. The result is the reinforcement of shame, guilt and condemnation; and feelings of abandonment and being alone.

1. _____
   _____
2. _____
   _____
3. _____
   _____

GROUP CHECK-IN

COMPLETE 24 HOURS BEFORE GROUP

1   What is the lowest level you reached on the *FASTER Scale* this week?

2   What was the *Double Bind* you were dealing with?

3   Where are you on your *Commitment to Change* from our last meeting?

4   Have you lied to anyone this week either directly or indirectly?

5   What have you done to improve your relationship with your wife or other significant relationships this week?

PILLAR FIVE
LESSON FOUR

CONSTRUCTING A WINNING BATTLE PLAN
WORKBOOK PAGE / 181

- [ ] Pillar Five: Lesson Four Video
- [ ] Workbook Assignment
- [ ] *Pure Desire* Reading
- [ ] Commitment to Change
- [ ] Devotional
- [ ] FASTER Scale
- [ ] Group Check-in

+ **Read Chapter 14 in *Pure Desire*. What were your observations?**

COMMITMENT TO CHANGE

1   What area do you need to change or what challenge are you facing next week?

2   What will it cost you emotionally if you do change? What fear will you have to face?

3   What will it cost you if you don't change?

4   What is your plan to maintain your restoration regarding these changes?

5   Who will you be accountable to as you pursue this commitment?

6   What are the details of this commitment? What information will you share with your accountability team when you touch base with them this week?

DEVOTIONAL

*³² "Now then, my children, listen to me;
blessed are those who keep my ways.
³³ Listen to my instruction and be wise;
do not disregard it.
³⁴ Blessed are those who listen to me,
watching daily at my doors,
waiting at my doorway.
³⁵ For those who find me find life
and receive favor from the Lord.
³⁶ But those who fail to find me harm themselves;
all who hate me love death."*

PROVERBS 8:32-36

 Read Proverbs 8.

SWORD DRILL

S **cripture** - Which verse or group of verses stood out to you in the Proverbs reading? Write it/them below.

W **ait** - Take a few moments now to wait on the Holy Spirit. Put aside any thoughts and worries of the day. Meditate on the Scripture. Read the verse(s) above aloud, slowly and attentively. Then pause to let it sink in. Let the Holy Spirit speak to you.

O **bserve** - What did you notice about the verse(s) from above? Was there something that the Holy Spirit spoke to you? Write your observation below.

R **equest** - Ask God to show you where and how the Scripture and observation apply to your life. Write the application below.

D **edicate Yourself** - Looking at how the Scripture applies to you, what is one thing that needs to change? Remember, this is not necessarily about something you need to do (or stop doing). Perhaps the change is in the way you see yourself or others.

FASTER SCALE

Adapted with permission from *The Genesis Process* by Michael Dye.

- ✦ **Circle the behaviors that you identify with in each section.**
- ✦ **Identify the most powerful behavior in each section and write it next to the corresponding heading.**
- ✦ **Answer the following three questions:**
    1. How does it affect me? How do I feel in the moment?
    2. How does it affect the important people in my life?
    3. Why do I do this? What is the benefit for me?

RESTORATION _____

(Accepting life on God's terms, with trust, grace, mercy, vulnerability and gratitude.)
No current secrets; working to resolve problems; identifying fears and feelings; keeping commitments to meetings, prayer, family, church, people, goals, and self; being open and honest, making eye contact; increasing in relationships with God and others; true accountability.

1. _____
2. _____
3. _____

FORGETTING PRIORITIES _____

(Start believing the present circumstances and moving away from trusting God. Denial; flight; a change in what's important; how you spend your time, energy, and thoughts.)
Secrets; less time/energy for God, meetings, church; avoiding support and accountability people; superficial conversations; sarcasm; isolating; changes in goals; obsessed with relationships; breaking promises and commitments; neglecting family; preoccupation with material things, TV, computers, entertainment; procrastination; lying; overconfidence; bored; hiding money; image management; seeking to control situations and other people.

1. _____
   _____
2. _____
   _____
3. _____
   _____

ANXIETY

(A growing background noise of undefined fear; getting energy from emotions.) Worry, using profanity, being fearful; being resentful; replaying old, negative thoughts; perfectionism; judging other's motives; making goals and lists that you can't complete; mind reading; fantasy, codependent rescuing; sleep problems, trouble concentrating, seeking/creating drama; gossip; using over-the-counter medication for pain, sleep or weight control; flirting.

1. _____
   _____
2. _____
   _____
3. _____
   _____

SPEEDING UP

(Trying to outrun the anxiety which is usually the first sign of depression.) Super busy and always in a hurry (finding good reason to justify the work); workaholic; can't relax; avoiding slowing down; feeling driven; can't turn off thoughts; skipping meals; binge eating (usually at night); overspending; can't identify own feelings/needs; repetitive negative thoughts; irritable; dramatic mood swings; too much caffeine; over exercising; nervousness; difficulty being alone and/or with people; difficulty listening to others; making excuses for having to "do it all."

1. _____
   _____
2. _____
   _____
3. _____
   _____

TICKED OFF

(Getting adrenaline high on anger and aggression.) Procrastination causing crisis in money, work, and relationships; increased sarcasm; black and white (all or nothing) thinking; feeling alone; nobody understands; overreacting, road rage; constant resentments; pushing others away; increasing isolation; blaming; arguing; irrational thinking; can't take criticism; defensive; people avoiding you; needing to be right; digestive problems; headaches; obsessive (stuck) thoughts; can't forgive; feeling superior; using intimidation.

1. _____
   _____
2. _____
   _____
3. _____
   _____

EXHAUSTED _____

(Loss of physical and emotional energy; coming off the adrenaline high, and the onset of depression.) Depressed; panicked; confused; hopelessness; sleeping too much or too little; can't cope; overwhelmed; crying for "no reason"; can't think; forgetful; pessimistic; helpless; tired; numb; wanting to run; constant cravings for old coping behaviors; thinking of using sex, drugs, or alcohol; seeking old unhealthy people and places; really isolating; people angry with you; self abuse; suicidal thoughts; spontaneous crying; no goals; survival mode; not returning phone calls; missing work; irritability; no appetite.

1. _____
   _____
2. _____
   _____
3. _____
   _____

RELAPSE _____

(Returning to the place you swore you would never go again. Coping with life on your terms. You sitting in the driver's seat instead of God.) Giving up and giving in; out of control; lost in your addiction; lying to yourself and others; feeling you just can't manage without your coping behaviors, at least for now. The result is the reinforcement of shame, guilt and condemnation; and feelings of abandonment and being alone.

1. _____
   _____
2. _____
   _____
3. _____
   _____

GROUP CHECK-IN

COMPLETE 24 HOURS BEFORE GROUP

1 What is the lowest level you reached on the *FASTER Scale* this week?

2 What was the *Double Bind* you were dealing with?

3 Where are you on your *Commitment to Change* from our last meeting?

4 Have you lied to anyone this week either directly or indirectly?

5 What have you done to improve your relationship with your wife or other significant relationships this week?

PILLAR SIX
LESSON ONE

MIGS COMING OUT OF THE WEEDS

WORKBOOK PAGE / 194

- [ ] Pillar Six Intro Video
- [ ] Pillar Six: Lesson One Video
- [ ] Workbook Assignment
- [ ] Commitment to Change
- [ ] Devotional
- [ ] FASTER Scale
- [ ] Group Check-in

COMMITMENT TO CHANGE

1 What area do you need to change or what challenge are you facing next week?

2 What will it cost you emotionally if you do change? What fear will you have to face?

3 What will it cost you if you don't change?

4 What is your plan to maintain your restoration regarding these changes?

5 Who will you be accountable to as you pursue this commitment?

6 What are the details of this commitment? What information will you share with your accountability team when you touch base with them this week?

DEVOTIONAL

> *[11] The house of the wicked will be destroyed,*
> *but the tent of the upright will flourish.*
>
> *[12] There is a way that appears to be right,*
> *but in the end it leads to death.*
>
> *[13] Even in laughter the heart may ache,*
> *and rejoicing may end in grief.*
>
> *[14] The faithless will be fully repaid for their ways,*
> *and the good rewarded for theirs.*
>
> *[15] The simple believe anything,*
> *but the prudent give thought to their steps.*
>
> *[16] The wise fear the Lord and shun evil,*
> *but a fool is hotheaded and yet feels secure.*
>
> *[17] A quick-tempered person does foolish things,*
> *and the one who devises evil schemes is hated.*
>
> *[18] The simple inherit folly,*
> *but the prudent are crowned with knowledge.*
>
> PROVERBS 14:11-18

 Read Proverbs 14.

SWORD DRILL

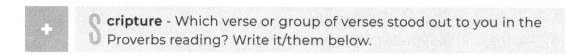

Scripture - Which verse or group of verses stood out to you in the Proverbs reading? Write it/them below.

Wait - Take a few moments now to wait on the Holy Spirit. Put aside any thoughts and worries of the day. Meditate on the Scripture. Read the verse(s) above aloud, slowly and attentively. Then pause to let it sink in. Let the Holy Spirit speak to you.

Observe - What did you notice about the verse(s) from above? Was there something that the Holy Spirit spoke to you? Write your observation below.

Request - Ask God to show you where and how the Scripture and observation apply to your life. Write the application below.

Dedicate Yourself - Looking at how the Scripture applies to you, what is one thing that needs to change? Remember, this is not necessarily about something you need to do (or stop doing). Perhaps the change is in the way you see yourself or others.

FASTER SCALE

Adapted with permission from *The Genesis Process* by Michael Dye.

+ **Circle the behaviors that you identify with in each section.**

+ **Identify the most powerful behavior in each section and write it next to the corresponding heading.**

+ **Answer the following three questions:**

  1. How does it affect me? How do I feel in the moment?

  2. How does it affect the important people in my life?

  3. Why do I do this? What is the benefit for me?

RESTORATION _____

(Accepting life on God's terms, with trust, grace, mercy, vulnerability and gratitude.) No current secrets; working to resolve problems; identifying fears and feelings; keeping commitments to meetings, prayer, family, church, people, goals, and self; being open and honest, making eye contact; increasing in relationships with God and others; true accountability.

1. _____

2. _____

3. _____

FORGETTING PRIORITIES _____

(Start believing the present circumstances and moving away from trusting God. Denial; flight; a change in what's important; how you spend your time, energy, and thoughts.) Secrets; less time/energy for God, meetings, church; avoiding support and accountability people; superficial conversations; sarcasm; isolating; changes in goals; obsessed with relationships; breaking promises and commitments; neglecting family; preoccupation with material things, TV, computers, entertainment; procrastination; lying; overconfidence; bored; hiding money; image management; seeking to control situations and other people.

1. _____

   _____

2. _____

   _____

3. _____

   _____

ANXIETY

(A growing background noise of undefined fear; getting energy from emotions.)
Worry, using profanity, being fearful; being resentful; replaying old, negative
thoughts; perfectionism; judging other's motives; making goals and lists that you
can't complete; mind reading; fantasy, codependent rescuing; sleep problems,
trouble concentrating, seeking/creating drama; gossip; using over-the-counter
medication for pain, sleep or weight control; flirting.

1. _____
   _____
2. _____
   _____
3. _____
   _____

SPEEDING UP

(Trying to outrun the anxiety which is usually the first sign of depression.) Super
busy and always in a hurry (finding good reason to justify the work); workaholic; can't
relax; avoiding slowing down; feeling driven; can't turn off thoughts; skipping meals;
binge eating (usually at night); overspending; can't identify own feelings/needs;
repetitive negative thoughts; irritable; dramatic mood swings; too much caffeine; over
exercising; nervousness; difficulty being alone and/or with people; difficulty listening
to others; making excuses for having to "do it all."

1. _____
   _____
2. _____
   _____
3. _____
   _____

TICKED OFF

(Getting adrenaline high on anger and aggression.) Procrastination causing crisis in
money, work, and relationships; increased sarcasm; black and white (all or nothing)
thinking; feeling alone; nobody understands; overreacting, road rage; constant resentments;
pushing others away; increasing isolation; blaming; arguing; irrational thinking; can't
take criticism; defensive; people avoiding you; needing to be right; digestive problems;
headaches; obsessive (stuck) thoughts; can't forgive; feeling superior; using intimidation.

1. _____

   _____

2. _____

   _____

3. _____

   _____

EXHAUSTED _____

(Loss of physical and emotional energy; coming off the adrenaline high, and the onset of depression.) Depressed; panicked; confused; hopelessness; sleeping too much or too little; can't cope; overwhelmed; crying for "no reason"; can't think; forgetful; pessimistic; helpless; tired; numb; wanting to run; constant cravings for old coping behaviors; thinking of using sex, drugs, or alcohol; seeking old unhealthy people and places; really isolating; people angry with you; self abuse; suicidal thoughts; spontaneous crying; no goals; survival mode; not returning phone calls; missing work; irritability; no appetite.

1. _____

   _____

2. _____

   _____

3. _____

   _____

RELAPSE _____

(Returning to the place you swore you would never go again. Coping with life on your terms. You sitting in the driver's seat instead of God.) Giving up and giving in; out of control; lost in your addiction; lying to yourself and others; feeling you just can't manage without your coping behaviors, at least for now. The result is the reinforcement of shame, guilt and condemnation; and feelings of abandonment and being alone.

1. _____

   _____

2. _____

   _____

3. _____

   _____

GROUP CHECK-IN

COMPLETE 24 HOURS BEFORE GROUP

1   What is the lowest level you reached on the *FASTER Scale* this week?

2   What was the *Double Bind* you were dealing with?

3   Where are you on your *Commitment to Change* from our last meeting?

4   Have you lied to anyone this week either directly or indirectly?

5   What have you done to improve your relationship with your wife or other significant relationships this week?

PILLAR SIX
LESSON TWO

WORKBOOK PAGE / 204

- ☐ Pillar Six: Lesson Two Video
- ☐ Workbook Assignment
- ☐ *Pure Desire* Reading
- ☐ Commitment to Change
- ☐ Devotional
- ☐ FASTER Scale
- ☐ Group Check-in

+   **Read Chapter 15 in *Pure Desire*. What were your observations?**

COMMITMENT TO CHANGE

1 What area do you need to change or what challenge are you facing next week?

2 What will it cost you emotionally if you do change? What fear will you have to face?

3 What will it cost you if you don't change?

4 What is your plan to maintain your restoration regarding these changes?

5 Who will you be accountable to as you pursue this commitment?

6 What are the details of this commitment? What information will you share with your accountability team when you touch base with them this week?

DEVOTIONAL

¹² Apply your heart to instruction
and your ears to words of knowledge.

¹³ Do not withhold discipline from a child;
if you punish them with the rod, they will not die.
¹⁴ Punish them with the rod
and save them from death.

¹⁵ My son, if your heart is wise,
then my heart will be glad indeed;
¹⁶ my inmost being will rejoice
when your lips speak what is right.

¹⁷ Do not let your heart envy sinners,
but always be zealous for the fear of the Lord.
¹⁸ There is surely a future hope for you,
and your hope will not be cut off.

PROVERBS 23:12-18

 Read Proverbs 23.

SWORD DRILL

S **cripture** - Which verse or group of verses stood out to you in the Proverbs reading? Write it/them below.

W **ait** - Take a few moments now to wait on the Holy Spirit. Put aside any thoughts and worries of the day. Meditate on the Scripture. Read the verse(s) above aloud, slowly and attentively. Then pause to let it sink in. Let the Holy Spirit speak to you.

O **bserve** - What did you notice about the verse(s) from above? Was there something that the Holy Spirit spoke to you? Write your observation below.

R **equest** - Ask God to show you where and how the Scripture and observation apply to your life. Write the application below.

D **edicate Yourself** - Looking at how the Scripture applies to you, what is one thing that needs to change? Remember, this is not necessarily about something you need to do (or stop doing). Perhaps the change is in the way you see yourself or others.

FASTER SCALE

Adapted with permission from *The Genesis Process* by Michael Dye.

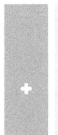

- ✦ **Circle the behaviors that you identify with in each section.**
- ✦ **Identify the most powerful behavior in each section and write it next to the corresponding heading.**
- ✦ **Answer the following three questions:**
  1. How does it affect me? How do I feel in the moment?
  2. How does it affect the important people in my life?
  3. Why do I do this? What is the benefit for me?

RESTORATION _____

(Accepting life on God's terms, with trust, grace, mercy, vulnerability and gratitude.) No current secrets; working to resolve problems; identifying fears and feelings; keeping commitments to meetings, prayer, family, church, people, goals, and self; being open and honest, making eye contact; increasing in relationships with God and others; true accountability.

1. _____
2. _____
3. _____

FORGETTING PRIORITIES _____

(Start believing the present circumstances and moving away from trusting God. Denial; flight; a change in what's important; how you spend your time, energy, and thoughts.) Secrets; less time/energy for God, meetings, church; avoiding support and accountability people; superficial conversations; sarcasm; isolating; changes in goals; obsessed with relationships; breaking promises and commitments; neglecting family; preoccupation with material things, TV, computers, entertainment; procrastination; lying; overconfidence; bored; hiding money; image management; seeking to control situations and other people.

1. _____
   _____
2. _____
   _____
3. _____
   _____

ANXIETY

(A growing background noise of undefined fear; getting energy from emotions.) Worry, using profanity, being fearful; being resentful; replaying old, negative thoughts; perfectionism; judging other's motives; making goals and lists that you can't complete; mind reading; fantasy, codependent rescuing; sleep problems, trouble concentrating, seeking/creating drama; gossip; using over-the-counter medication for pain, sleep or weight control; flirting.

1. _____
   _____

2. _____
   _____

3. _____
   _____

SPEEDING UP

(Trying to outrun the anxiety which is usually the first sign of depression.) Super busy and always in a hurry (finding good reason to justify the work); workaholic; can't relax; avoiding slowing down; feeling driven; can't turn off thoughts; skipping meals; binge eating (usually at night); overspending; can't identify own feelings/needs; repetitive negative thoughts; irritable; dramatic mood swings; too much caffeine; over exercising; nervousness; difficulty being alone and/or with people; difficulty listening to others; making excuses for having to "do it all."

1. _____
   _____

2. _____
   _____

3. _____
   _____

TICKED OFF

(Getting adrenaline high on anger and aggression.) Procrastination causing crisis in money, work, and relationships; increased sarcasm; black and white (all or nothing) thinking; feeling alone; nobody understands; overreacting, road rage; constant resentments; pushing others away; increasing isolation; blaming; arguing; irrational thinking; can't take criticism; defensive; people avoiding you; needing to be right; digestive problems; headaches; obsessive (stuck) thoughts; can't forgive; feeling superior; using intimidation.

1. _____

_____

2. _____

_____

3. _____

_____

EXHAUSTED _____

(Loss of physical and emotional energy; coming off the adrenaline high, and the onset of depression.) Depressed; panicked; confused; hopelessness; sleeping too much or too little; can't cope; overwhelmed; crying for "no reason"; can't think; forgetful; pessimistic; helpless; tired; numb; wanting to run; constant cravings for old coping behaviors; thinking of using sex, drugs, or alcohol; seeking old unhealthy people and places; really isolating; people angry with you; self abuse; suicidal thoughts; spontaneous crying; no goals; survival mode; not returning phone calls; missing work; irritability; no appetite.

1. _____

_____

2. _____

_____

3. _____

_____

RELAPSE _____

(Returning to the place you swore you would never go again. Coping with life on your terms. You sitting in the driver's seat instead of God.) Giving up and giving in; out of control; lost in your addiction; lying to yourself and others; feeling you just can't manage without your coping behaviors, at least for now. The result is the reinforcement of shame, guilt and condemnation; and feelings of abandonment and being alone.

1. _____

_____

2. _____

_____

3. _____

_____

GROUP CHECK-IN

COMPLETE 24 HOURS BEFORE GROUP

1   What is the lowest level you reached on the *FASTER Scale* this week?

2   What was the *Double Bind* you were dealing with?

3   Where are you on your *Commitment to Change* from our last meeting?

4   Have you lied to anyone this week either directly or indirectly?

5   What have you done to improve your relationship with your wife or other significant relationships this week?

PILLAR SIX
LESSON THREE

LEARNING TO TURN INTO THE FIGHT
WORKBOOK PAGE / 215

- ☐ Pillar Six: Lesson Three Video
- ☐ Workbook Assignment
- ☐ Commitment to Change
- ☐ Devotional
- ☐ FASTER Scale
- ☐ Group Check-in

COMMITMENT TO CHANGE

1   What area do you need to change or what challenge are you facing next week?

2   What will it cost you emotionally if you do change? What fear will you have to face?

3   What will it cost you if you don't change?

4   What is your plan to maintain your restoration regarding these changes?

5   Who will you be accountable to as you pursue this commitment?

6   What are the details of this commitment? What information will you share with your accountability team when you touch base with them this week?

DEVOTIONAL

⁵ The plans of the righteous are just,
but the advice of the wicked is deceitful.

⁶ The words of the wicked lie in wait for blood,
but the speech of the upright rescues them.

⁷ The wicked are overthrown and are no more,
but the house of the righteous stands firm.

⁸ A person is praised according to their prudence,
and one with a warped mind is despised.

⁹ Better to be a nobody and yet have a servant
than pretend to be somebody and have no food.

¹⁰ The righteous care for the needs of their animals,
but the kindest acts of the wicked are cruel.

¹¹ Those who work their land will have abundant food,
but those who chase fantasies have no sense.

¹² The wicked desire the stronghold of evildoers,
but the root of the righteous endures.

PROVERBS 12:5-12

 Read Proverbs 12.

SWORD DRILL

S **cripture** - Which verse or group of verses stood out to you in the Proverbs reading? Write it/them below.

W **ait** - Take a few moments now to wait on the Holy Spirit. Put aside any thoughts and worries of the day. Meditate on the Scripture. Read the verse(s) above aloud, slowly and attentively. Then pause to let it sink in. Let the Holy Spirit speak to you.

O **bserve** - What did you notice about the verse(s) from above? Was there something that the Holy Spirit spoke to you? Write your observation below.

R **equest** - Ask God to show you where and how the Scripture and observation apply to your life. Write the application below.

D **edicate Yourself** - Looking at how the Scripture applies to you, what is one thing that needs to change? Remember, this is not necessarily about something you need to do (or stop doing). Perhaps the change is in the way you see yourself or others.

FASTER SCALE

Adapted with permission from *The Genesis Process* by Michael Dye.

- Circle the behaviors that you identify with in each section.
- Identify the most powerful behavior in each section and write it next to the corresponding heading.
- Answer the following three questions:
  1. How does it affect me? How do I feel in the moment?
  2. How does it affect the important people in my life?
  3. Why do I do this? What is the benefit for me?

RESTORATION _____

(Accepting life on God's terms, with trust, grace, mercy, vulnerability and gratitude.) No current secrets; working to resolve problems; identifying fears and feelings; keeping commitments to meetings, prayer, family, church, people, goals, and self; being open and honest, making eye contact; increasing in relationships with God and others; true accountability.

1. _____
2. _____
3. _____

FORGETTING PRIORITIES _____

(Start believing the present circumstances and moving away from trusting God. Denial; flight; a change in what's important; how you spend your time, energy, and thoughts.) Secrets; less time/energy for God, meetings, church; avoiding support and accountability people; superficial conversations; sarcasm; isolating; changes in goals; obsessed with relationships; breaking promises and commitments; neglecting family; preoccupation with material things, TV, computers, entertainment; procrastination; lying; overconfidence; bored; hiding money; image management; seeking to control situations and other people.

1. _____
   _____
2. _____
   _____
3. _____
   _____

ANXIETY

(A growing background noise of undefined fear; getting energy from emotions.) Worry, using profanity, being fearful; being resentful; replaying old, negative thoughts; perfectionism; judging other's motives; making goals and lists that you can't complete; mind reading; fantasy, codependent rescuing; sleep problems, trouble concentrating, seeking/creating drama; gossip; using over-the-counter medication for pain, sleep or weight control; flirting.

1. _____
_____

2. _____
_____

3. _____
_____

SPEEDING UP

(Trying to outrun the anxiety which is usually the first sign of depression.) Super busy and always in a hurry (finding good reason to justify the work); workaholic; can't relax; avoiding slowing down; feeling driven; can't turn off thoughts; skipping meals; binge eating (usually at night); overspending; can't identify own feelings/needs; repetitive negative thoughts; irritable; dramatic mood swings; too much caffeine; over exercising; nervousness; difficulty being alone and/or with people; difficulty listening to others; making excuses for having to "do it all."

1. _____
_____

2. _____
_____

3. _____
_____

TICKED OFF

(Getting adrenaline high on anger and aggression.) Procrastination causing crisis in money, work, and relationships; increased sarcasm; black and white (all or nothing) thinking; feeling alone; nobody understands; overreacting, road rage; constant resentments; pushing others away; increasing isolation; blaming; arguing; irrational thinking; can't take criticism; defensive; people avoiding you; needing to be right; digestive problems; headaches; obsessive (stuck) thoughts; can't forgive; feeling superior; using intimidation.

1. _____

_____

2. _____

_____

3. _____

_____

EXHAUSTED _____

(Loss of physical and emotional energy; coming off the adrenaline high, and the onset of depression.) Depressed; panicked; confused; hopelessness; sleeping too much or too little; can't cope; overwhelmed; crying for "no reason"; can't think; forgetful; pessimistic; helpless; tired; numb; wanting to run; constant cravings for old coping behaviors; thinking of using sex, drugs, or alcohol; seeking old unhealthy people and places; really isolating; people angry with you; self abuse; suicidal thoughts; spontaneous crying; no goals; survival mode; not returning phone calls; missing work; irritability; no appetite.

1. _____

_____

2. _____

_____

3. _____

_____

RELAPSE _____

(Returning to the place you swore you would never go again. Coping with life on your terms. You sitting in the driver's seat instead of God.) Giving up and giving in; out of control; lost in your addiction; lying to yourself and others; feeling you just can't manage without your coping behaviors, at least for now. The result is the reinforcement of shame, guilt and condemnation; and feelings of abandonment and being alone.

1. _____

_____

2. _____

_____

3. _____

_____

GROUP CHECK-IN

COMPLETE 24 HOURS BEFORE GROUP

1   What is the lowest level you reached on the *FASTER Scale* this week?

2   What was the *Double Bind* you were dealing with?

3   Where are you on your *Commitment to Change* from our last meeting?

4   Have you lied to anyone this week either directly or indirectly?

5   What have you done to improve your relationship with your wife or other significant relationships this week?

PILLAR SIX
LESSON FOUR

POWER TOOLS
WORKBOOK PAGE / 230

- ☐ Pillar Six: Lesson Four Video
- ☐ Workbook Assignment
- ☐ Commitment to Change
- ☐ Devotional
- ☐ FASTER Scale
- ☐ Group Check-in

COMMITMENT TO CHANGE

1   What area do you need to change or what challenge are you facing next week?

2   What will it cost you emotionally if you do change? What fear will you have to face?

3   What will it cost you if you don't change?

4   What is your plan to maintain your restoration regarding these changes?

5   Who will you be accountable to as you pursue this commitment?

6   What are the details of this commitment? What information will you share with your accountability team when you touch base with them this week?

DEVOTIONAL

*⁴ Remove the dross from the silver,
and a silversmith can produce a vessel;
⁵ remove wicked officials from the king's presence,
and his throne will be established through righteousness.*

*⁶ Do not exalt yourself in the king's presence,
and do not claim a place among his great men;
⁷ it is better for him to say to you, "Come up here,"
than for him to humiliate you before his nobles.*

*What you have seen with your eyes
⁸ do not bring hastily to court,
for what will you do in the end
if your neighbor puts you to shame?*

*⁹ If you take your neighbor to court,
do not betray another's confidence,
¹⁰ or the one who hears it may shame you
and the charge against you will stand.*

*¹¹ Like apples of gold in settings of silver
is a ruling rightly given.
¹² Like an earring of gold or an ornament of fine gold
is the rebuke of a wise judge to a listening ear.*

PROVERBS 25:4-12

 Read Proverbs 25.

SWORD DRILL

Scripture - Which verse or group of verses stood out to you in the Proverbs reading? Write it/them below.

Wait - Take a few moments now to wait on the Holy Spirit. Put aside any thoughts and worries of the day. Meditate on the Scripture. Read the verse(s) above aloud, slowly and attentively. Then pause to let it sink in. Let the Holy Spirit speak to you.

Observe - What did you notice about the verse(s) from above? Was there something that the Holy Spirit spoke to you? Write your observation below.

Request - Ask God to show you where and how the Scripture and observation apply to your life. Write the application below.

Dedicate Yourself - Looking at how the Scripture applies to you, what is one thing that needs to change? Remember, this is not necessarily about something you need to do (or stop doing). Perhaps the change is in the way you see yourself or others.

FASTER SCALE

Adapted with permission from *The Genesis Process* by Michael Dye.

- Circle the behaviors that you identify with in each section.
- Identify the most powerful behavior in each section and write it next to the corresponding heading.
- Answer the following three questions:
  1. How does it affect me? How do I feel in the moment?
  2. How does it affect the important people in my life?
  3. Why do I do this? What is the benefit for me?

RESTORATION _____

(Accepting life on God's terms, with trust, grace, mercy, vulnerability and gratitude.)
No current secrets; working to resolve problems; identifying fears and feelings; keeping commitments to meetings, prayer, family, church, people, goals, and self; being open and honest, making eye contact; increasing in relationships with God and others; true accountability.

1. _____
2. _____
3. _____

FORGETTING PRIORITIES _____

(Start believing the present circumstances and moving away from trusting God. Denial; flight; a change in what's important; how you spend your time, energy, and thoughts.)
Secrets; less time/energy for God, meetings, church; avoiding support and accountability people; superficial conversations; sarcasm; isolating; changes in goals; obsessed with relationships; breaking promises and commitments; neglecting family; preoccupation with material things, TV, computers, entertainment; procrastination; lying; overconfidence; bored; hiding money; image management; seeking to control situations and other people.

1. _____
   _____
2. _____
   _____
3. _____
   _____

ANXIETY

(A growing background noise of undefined fear; getting energy from emotions.)
Worry, using profanity, being fearful; being resentful; replaying old, negative thoughts; perfectionism; judging other's motives; making goals and lists that you can't complete; mind reading; fantasy, codependent rescuing; sleep problems, trouble concentrating, seeking/creating drama; gossip; using over-the-counter medication for pain, sleep or weight control; flirting.

1. _____
   _____
2. _____
   _____
3. _____
   _____

SPEEDING UP

(Trying to outrun the anxiety which is usually the first sign of depression.) Super busy and always in a hurry (finding good reason to justify the work); workaholic; can't relax; avoiding slowing down; feeling driven; can't turn off thoughts; skipping meals; binge eating (usually at night); overspending; can't identify own feelings/needs; repetitive negative thoughts; irritable; dramatic mood swings; too much caffeine; over exercising; nervousness; difficulty being alone and/or with people; difficulty listening to others; making excuses for having to "do it all."

1. _____
   _____
2. _____
   _____
3. _____
   _____

TICKED OFF

(Getting adrenaline high on anger and aggression.) Procrastination causing crisis in money, work, and relationships; increased sarcasm; black and white (all or nothing) thinking; feeling alone; nobody understands; overreacting, road rage; constant resentments; pushing others away; increasing isolation; blaming; arguing; irrational thinking; can't take criticism; defensive; people avoiding you; needing to be right; digestive problems; headaches; obsessive (stuck) thoughts; can't forgive; feeling superior; using intimidation.

1. _____

_____

2. _____

_____

3. _____

_____

EXHAUSTED _____

(Loss of physical and emotional energy; coming off the adrenaline high, and the onset of depression.) Depressed; panicked; confused; hopelessness; sleeping too much or too little; can't cope; overwhelmed; crying for "no reason"; can't think; forgetful; pessimistic; helpless; tired; numb; wanting to run; constant cravings for old coping behaviors; thinking of using sex, drugs, or alcohol; seeking old unhealthy people and places; really isolating; people angry with you; self abuse; suicidal thoughts; spontaneous crying; no goals; survival mode; not returning phone calls; missing work; irritability; no appetite.

1. _____

_____

2. _____

_____

3. _____

_____

RELAPSE _____

(Returning to the place you swore you would never go again. Coping with life on your terms. You sitting in the driver's seat instead of God.) Giving up and giving in; out of control; lost in your addiction; lying to yourself and others; feeling you just can't manage without your coping behaviors, at least for now. The result is the reinforcement of shame, guilt and condemnation; and feelings of abandonment and being alone.

1. _____

_____

2. _____

_____

3. _____

_____

GROUP CHECK-IN

COMPLETE 24 HOURS BEFORE GROUP

1   What is the lowest level you reached on the *FASTER Scale* this week?

2   What was the *Double Bind* you were dealing with?

3   Where are you on your *Commitment to Change* from our last meeting?

4   Have you lied to anyone this week either directly or indirectly?

5   What have you done to improve your relationship with your wife or other significant relationships this week?

PILLAR SEVEN
LESSON ONE

DISCLOSURE
WORKBOOK PAGE / 248

☐ Pillar Seven Intro Video

☐ Pillar Seven: Lesson One Video

☐ Workbook Assignment

☐ *Pure Desire* Reading

☐ Commitment to Change

☐ Devotional

☐ FASTER Scale

☐ Group Check-in

+ **Read Chapter 16 in *Pure Desire*. What were your observations?**

COMMITMENT TO CHANGE

1 What area do you need to change or what challenge are you facing next week?

2 What will it cost you emotionally if you do change? What fear will you have to face?

3 What will it cost you if you don't change?

4 What is your plan to maintain your restoration regarding these changes?

5 Who will you be accountable to as you pursue this commitment?

6 What are the details of this commitment? What information will you share with your accountability team when you touch base with them this week?

DEVOTIONAL

⁵ Every word of God is flawless;
he is a shield to those who take refuge in him.
⁶ Do not add to his words,
or he will rebuke you and prove you a liar.

⁷ Two things I ask of you, Lord;
do not refuse me before I die:
⁸ Keep falsehood and lies far from me;
give me neither poverty nor riches,
but give me only my daily bread.
⁹ Otherwise, I may have too much and disown you
and say, 'Who is the Lord?'
Or I may become poor and steal,
and so dishonor the name of my God.

PROVERBS 30:5-9

 Read Proverbs 30.

SWORD DRILL

S **cripture** - Which verse or group of verses stood out to you in the Proverbs reading? Write it/them below.

W **ait** - Take a few moments now to wait on the Holy Spirit. Put aside any thoughts and worries of the day. Meditate on the Scripture. Read the verse(s) above aloud, slowly and attentively. Then pause to let it sink in. Let the Holy Spirit speak to you.

O **bserve** - What did you notice about the verse(s) from above? Was there something that the Holy Spirit spoke to you? Write your observation below.

R **equest** - Ask God to show you where and how the Scripture and observation apply to your life. Write the application below.

D **edicate Yourself** - Looking at how the Scripture applies to you, what is one thing that needs to change? Remember, this is not necessarily about something you need to do (or stop doing). Perhaps the change is in the way you see yourself or others.

FASTER SCALE

Adapted with permission from *The Genesis Process* by Michael Dye.

- Circle the behaviors that you identify with in each section.
- Identify the most powerful behavior in each section and write it next to the corresponding heading.
- Answer the following three questions:
  1. How does it affect me? How do I feel in the moment?
  2. How does it affect the important people in my life?
  3. Why do I do this? What is the benefit for me?

RESTORATION _____

(Accepting life on God's terms, with trust, grace, mercy, vulnerability and gratitude.)
No current secrets; working to resolve problems; identifying fears and feelings; keeping commitments to meetings, prayer, family, church, people, goals, and self; being open and honest, making eye contact; increasing in relationships with God and others; true accountability.

1. _____
2. _____
3. _____

FORGETTING PRIORITIES _____

(Start believing the present circumstances and moving away from trusting God. Denial; flight; a change in what's important; how you spend your time, energy, and thoughts.)
Secrets; less time/energy for God, meetings, church; avoiding support and accountability people; superficial conversations; sarcasm; isolating; changes in goals; obsessed with relationships; breaking promises and commitments; neglecting family; preoccupation with material things, TV, computers, entertainment; procrastination; lying; overconfidence; bored; hiding money; image management; seeking to control situations and other people.

1. _____
   _____
2. _____
   _____
3. _____
   _____

ANXIETY

(A growing background noise of undefined fear; getting energy from emotions.) Worry, using profanity, being fearful; being resentful; replaying old, negative thoughts; perfectionism; judging other's motives; making goals and lists that you can't complete; mind reading; fantasy, codependent rescuing; sleep problems, trouble concentrating, seeking/creating drama; gossip; using over-the-counter medication for pain, sleep or weight control; flirting.

1. _____
   _____
2. _____
   _____
3. _____
   _____

SPEEDING UP

(Trying to outrun the anxiety which is usually the first sign of depression.) Super busy and always in a hurry (finding good reason to justify the work); workaholic; can't relax; avoiding slowing down; feeling driven; can't turn off thoughts; skipping meals; binge eating (usually at night); overspending; can't identify own feelings/needs; repetitive negative thoughts; irritable; dramatic mood swings; too much caffeine; over exercising; nervousness; difficulty being alone and/or with people; difficulty listening to others; making excuses for having to "do it all."

1. _____
   _____
2. _____
   _____
3. _____
   _____

TICKED OFF

(Getting adrenaline high on anger and aggression.) Procrastination causing crisis in money, work, and relationships; increased sarcasm; black and white (all or nothing) thinking; feeling alone; nobody understands; overreacting, road rage; constant resentments; pushing others away; increasing isolation; blaming; arguing; irrational thinking; can't take criticism; defensive; people avoiding you; needing to be right; digestive problems; headaches; obsessive (stuck) thoughts; can't forgive; feeling superior; using intimidation.

1. _____

2. _____

3. _____

EXHAUSTED _____

(Loss of physical and emotional energy; coming off the adrenaline high, and the onset of depression.) Depressed; panicked; confused; hopelessness; sleeping too much or too little; can't cope; overwhelmed; crying for "no reason"; can't think; forgetful; pessimistic; helpless; tired; numb; wanting to run; constant cravings for old coping behaviors; thinking of using sex, drugs, or alcohol; seeking old unhealthy people and places; really isolating; people angry with you; self abuse; suicidal thoughts; spontaneous crying; no goals; survival mode; not returning phone calls; missing work; irritability; no appetite.

1. _____

2. _____

3. _____

RELAPSE _____

(Returning to the place you swore you would never go again. Coping with life on your terms. You sitting in the driver's seat instead of God.) Giving up and giving in; out of control; lost in your addiction; lying to yourself and others; feeling you just can't manage without your coping behaviors, at least for now. The result is the reinforcement of shame, guilt and condemnation; and feelings of abandonment and being alone.

1. _____

2. _____

3. _____

GROUP CHECK-IN

COMPLETE 24 HOURS BEFORE GROUP

1   What is the lowest level you reached on the *FASTER Scale* this week?

2   What was the *Double Bind* you were dealing with?

3   Where are you on your *Commitment to Change* from our last meeting?

4   Have you lied to anyone this week either directly or indirectly?

5   What have you done to improve your relationship with your wife or other significant relationships this week?

PILLAR SEVEN
LESSON TWO

HELPING YOUR WIFE MOVE THROUGH HER HEALING TO HEALTHY SEXUALITY (PART ONE)

WORKBOOK PAGE / 256

- [ ] Pillar Seven: Lesson Two Video
- [ ] Workbook Assignment
- [ ] Commitment to Change
- [ ] Devotional
- [ ] FASTER Scale
- [ ] Group Check-in

COMMITMENT TO CHANGE

1   What area do you need to change or what challenge are you facing next week?

2   What will it cost you emotionally if you do change? What fear will you have to face?

3   What will it cost you if you don't change?

4   What is your plan to maintain your restoration regarding these changes?

5   Who will you be accountable to as you pursue this commitment?

6   What are the details of this commitment? What information will you share with your accountability team when you touch base with them this week?

DEVOTIONAL

23 Her husband is respected at the city gate,
where he takes his seat among the elders of the land.
24 She makes linen garments and sells them,
and supplies the merchants with sashes.
25 She is clothed with strength and dignity;
she can laugh at the days to come.
26 She speaks with wisdom,
and faithful instruction is on her tongue.
27 She watches over the affairs of her household
and does not eat the bread of idleness.
28 Her children arise and call her blessed;
her husband also, and he praises her:
29 "Many women do noble things,
but you surpass them all."
30 Charm is deceptive, and beauty is fleeting;
but a woman who fears the Lord is to be praised.
31 Honor her for all that her hands have done,
and let her works bring her praise at the city gate.

PROVERBS 31:23-31

 Read Proverbs 31.

SWORD DRILL

S **cripture** - Which verse or group of verses stood out to you in the Proverbs reading? Write it/them below.

W **ait** - Take a few moments now to wait on the Holy Spirit. Put aside any thoughts and worries of the day. Meditate on the Scripture. Read the verse(s) above aloud, slowly and attentively. Then pause to let it sink in. Let the Holy Spirit speak to you.

O **bserve** - What did you notice about the verse(s) from above? Was there something that the Holy Spirit spoke to you? Write your observation below.

R **equest** - Ask God to show you where and how the Scripture and observation apply to your life. Write the application below.

D **edicate Yourself** - Looking at how the Scripture applies to you, what is one thing that needs to change? Remember, this is not necessarily about something you need to do (or stop doing). Perhaps the change is in the way you see yourself or others.

FASTER SCALE

Adapted with permission from *The Genesis Process* by Michael Dye.

- Circle the behaviors that you identify with in each section.
- Identify the most powerful behavior in each section and write it next to the corresponding heading.
- Answer the following three questions:
  1. How does it affect me? How do I feel in the moment?
  2. How does it affect the important people in my life?
  3. Why do I do this? What is the benefit for me?

RESTORATION _____

(Accepting life on God's terms, with trust, grace, mercy, vulnerability and gratitude.) No current secrets; working to resolve problems; identifying fears and feelings; keeping commitments to meetings, prayer, family, church, people, goals, and self; being open and honest, making eye contact; increasing in relationships with God and others; true accountability.

1. _____

2. _____

3. _____

FORGETTING PRIORITIES _____

(Start believing the present circumstances and moving away from trusting God. Denial; flight; a change in what's important; how you spend your time, energy, and thoughts.) Secrets; less time/energy for God, meetings, church; avoiding support and accountability people; superficial conversations; sarcasm; isolating; changes in goals; obsessed with relationships; breaking promises and commitments; neglecting family; preoccupation with material things, TV, computers, entertainment; procrastination; lying; overconfidence; bored; hiding money; image management; seeking to control situations and other people.

1. _____
   _____

2. _____
   _____

3. _____
   _____

ANXIETY

(A growing background noise of undefined fear; getting energy from emotions.)
Worry, using profanity, being fearful; being resentful; replaying old, negative
thoughts; perfectionism; judging other's motives; making goals and lists that you
can't complete; mind reading; fantasy, codependent rescuing; sleep problems,
trouble concentrating, seeking/creating drama; gossip; using over-the-counter
medication for pain, sleep or weight control; flirting.

1. _____

   _____

2. _____

   _____

3. _____

   _____

SPEEDING UP

(Trying to outrun the anxiety which is usually the first sign of depression.) Super
busy and always in a hurry (finding good reason to justify the work); workaholic; can't
relax; avoiding slowing down; feeling driven; can't turn off thoughts; skipping meals;
binge eating (usually at night); overspending; can't identify own feelings/needs;
repetitive negative thoughts; irritable; dramatic mood swings; too much caffeine; over
exercising; nervousness; difficulty being alone and/or with people; difficulty listening
to others; making excuses for having to "do it all."

1. _____

   _____

2. _____

   _____

3. _____

   _____

TICKED OFF

(Getting adrenaline high on anger and aggression.) Procrastination causing crisis in
money, work, and relationships; increased sarcasm; black and white (all or nothing)
thinking; feeling alone; nobody understands; overreacting, road rage; constant resentments;
pushing others away; increasing isolation; blaming; arguing; irrational thinking; can't
take criticism; defensive; people avoiding you; needing to be right; digestive problems;
headaches; obsessive (stuck) thoughts; can't forgive; feeling superior; using intimidation.

1. _____

   _____

2. _____

   _____

3. _____

   _____

EXHAUSTED

(Loss of physical and emotional energy; coming off the adrenaline high, and the onset of depression.) Depressed; panicked; confused; hopelessness; sleeping too much or too little; can't cope; overwhelmed; crying for "no reason"; can't think; forgetful; pessimistic; helpless; tired; numb; wanting to run; constant cravings for old coping behaviors; thinking of using sex, drugs, or alcohol; seeking old unhealthy people and places; really isolating; people angry with you; self abuse; suicidal thoughts; spontaneous crying; no goals; survival mode; not returning phone calls; missing work; irritability; no appetite.

1. _____

   _____

2. _____

   _____

3. _____

   _____

RELAPSE

(Returning to the place you swore you would never go again. Coping with life on your terms. You sitting in the driver's seat instead of God.) Giving up and giving in; out of control; lost in your addiction; lying to yourself and others; feeling you just can't manage without your coping behaviors, at least for now. The result is the reinforcement of shame, guilt and condemnation; and feelings of abandonment and being alone.

1. _____

   _____

2. _____

   _____

3. _____

   _____

GROUP CHECK-IN

COMPLETE 24 HOURS BEFORE GROUP

1   What is the lowest level you reached on the *FASTER Scale* this week?

2   What was the *Double Bind* you were dealing with?

3   Where are you on your *Commitment to Change* from our last meeting?

4   Have you lied to anyone this week either directly or indirectly?

5   What have you done to improve your relationship with your wife or other significant relationships this week?

HELPING YOUR WIFE MOVE THROUGH HER HEALING TO HEALTHY SEXUALITY (PART TWO)

WORKBOOK PAGE / 265

☐ Pillar Seven: Lesson Three Video

☐ Workbook Assignment

☐ Commitment to Change

☐ Devotional

☐ FASTER Scale

☐ Group Check-in

COMMITMENT TO CHANGE

1   What area do you need to change or what challenge are you facing next week?

2   What will it cost you emotionally if you do change? What fear will you have to face?

3   What will it cost you if you don't change?

4   What is your plan to maintain your restoration regarding these changes?

5   Who will you be accountable to as you pursue this commitment?

6   What are the details of this commitment? What information will you share with your accountability team when you touch base with them this week?

DEVOTIONAL

*¹¹ I instruct you in the way of wisdom
and lead you along straight paths.*
*¹² When you walk, your steps will not be hampered;
when you run, you will not stumble.*
*¹³ Hold on to instruction, do not let it go;
guard it well, for it is your life.*
*¹⁴ Do not set foot on the path of the wicked
or walk in the way of evildoers.*
*¹⁵ Avoid it, do not travel on it;
turn from it and go on your way.*
*¹⁶ For they cannot rest until they do evil;
they are robbed of sleep till they make someone stumble.*
*¹⁷ They eat the bread of wickedness
and drink the wine of violence.*

*¹⁸ The path of the righteous is like the morning sun,
shining ever brighter till the full light of day.*
*¹⁹ But the way of the wicked is like deep darkness;
they do not know what makes them stumble.*

PROVERBS 4:11-19

 Read Proverbs 4.

SWORD DRILL

S cripture - Which verse or group of verses stood out to you in the Proverbs reading? Write it/them below.

W ait - Take a few moments now to wait on the Holy Spirit. Put aside any thoughts and worries of the day. Meditate on the Scripture. Read the verse(s) above aloud, slowly and attentively. Then pause to let it sink in. Let the Holy Spirit speak to you.

O bserve - What did you notice about the verse(s) from above? Was there something that the Holy Spirit spoke to you? Write your observation below.

R equest - Ask God to show you where and how the Scripture and observation apply to your life. Write the application below.

D edicate Yourself - Looking at how the Scripture applies to you, what is one thing that needs to change? Remember, this is not necessarily about something you need to do (or stop doing). Perhaps the change is in the way you see yourself or others.

FASTER SCALE

Adapted with permission from *The Genesis Process* by Michael Dye.

- Circle the behaviors that you identify with in each section.
- Identify the most powerful behavior in each section and write it next to the corresponding heading.
- Answer the following three questions:
  1. How does it affect me? How do I feel in the moment?
  2. How does it affect the important people in my life?
  3. Why do I do this? What is the benefit for me?

RESTORATION _____

(Accepting life on God's terms, with trust, grace, mercy, vulnerability and gratitude.)
No current secrets; working to resolve problems; identifying fears and feelings; keeping commitments to meetings, prayer, family, church, people, goals, and self; being open and honest, making eye contact; increasing in relationships with God and others; true accountability.

1. _____
2. _____
3. _____

FORGETTING PRIORITIES _____

(Start believing the present circumstances and moving away from trusting God. Denial; flight; a change in what's important; how you spend your time, energy, and thoughts.)
Secrets; less time/energy for God, meetings, church; avoiding support and accountability people; superficial conversations; sarcasm; isolating; changes in goals; obsessed with relationships; breaking promises and commitments; neglecting family; preoccupation with material things, TV, computers, entertainment; procrastination; lying; overconfidence; bored; hiding money; image management; seeking to control situations and other people.

1. _____
   _____
2. _____
   _____
3. _____
   _____

ANXIETY

(A growing background noise of undefined fear; getting energy from emotions.)
Worry, using profanity, being fearful; being resentful; replaying old, negative
thoughts; perfectionism; judging other's motives; making goals and lists that you
can't complete; mind reading; fantasy, codependent rescuing; sleep problems,
trouble concentrating, seeking/creating drama; gossip; using over-the-counter
medication for pain, sleep or weight control; flirting.

1. _____
   _____

2. _____
   _____

3. _____
   _____

SPEEDING UP

(Trying to outrun the anxiety which is usually the first sign of depression.) Super
busy and always in a hurry (finding good reason to justify the work); workaholic; can't
relax; avoiding slowing down; feeling driven; can't turn off thoughts; skipping meals;
binge eating (usually at night); overspending; can't identify own feelings/needs;
repetitive negative thoughts; irritable; dramatic mood swings; too much caffeine; over
exercising; nervousness; difficulty being alone and/or with people; difficulty listening
to others; making excuses for having to "do it all."

1. _____
   _____

2. _____
   _____

3. _____
   _____

TICKED OFF

(Getting adrenaline high on anger and aggression.) Procrastination causing crisis in
money, work, and relationships; increased sarcasm; black and white (all or nothing)
thinking; feeling alone; nobody understands; overreacting, road rage; constant resentments;
pushing others away; increasing isolation; blaming; arguing; irrational thinking; can't
take criticism; defensive; people avoiding you; needing to be right; digestive problems;
headaches; obsessive (stuck) thoughts; can't forgive; feeling superior; using intimidation.

1. _____

2. _____

3. _____

EXHAUSTED _____

(Loss of physical and emotional energy; coming off the adrenaline high, and the onset of depression.) Depressed; panicked; confused; hopelessness; sleeping too much or too little; can't cope; overwhelmed; crying for "no reason"; can't think; forgetful; pessimistic; helpless; tired; numb; wanting to run; constant cravings for old coping behaviors; thinking of using sex, drugs, or alcohol; seeking old unhealthy people and places; really isolating; people angry with you; self abuse; suicidal thoughts; spontaneous crying; no goals; survival mode; not returning phone calls; missing work; irritability; no appetite.

1. _____

2. _____

3. _____

RELAPSE _____

(Returning to the place you swore you would never go again. Coping with life on your terms. You sitting in the driver's seat instead of God.) Giving up and giving in; out of control; lost in your addiction; lying to yourself and others; feeling you just can't manage without your coping behaviors, at least for now. The result is the reinforcement of shame, guilt and condemnation; and feelings of abandonment and being alone.

1. _____

2. _____

3. _____

GROUP CHECK-IN

COMPLETE 24 HOURS BEFORE GROUP

1   What is the lowest level you reached on the *FASTER Scale* this week?

2   What was the *Double Bind* you were dealing with?

3   Where are you on your *Commitment to Change* from our last meeting?

4   Have you lied to anyone this week either directly or indirectly?

5   What have you done to improve your relationship with your wife or other significant relationships this week?

PILLAR SEVEN
LESSON FOUR

SELF-CONTROL & VISION
WORKBOOK PAGE / 274

- ☐ Pillar Seven: Lesson Four Video
- ☐ Workbook Assignment
- ☐ *Pure Desire* Reading
- ☐ Commitment to Change
- ☐ Devotional
- ☐ FASTER Scale
- ☐ Group Check-in

+   **Read Chapter 17 in *Pure Desire*. What were your observations?**

COMMITMENT TO CHANGE

1   What area do you need to change or what challenge are you facing next week?

2   What will it cost you emotionally if you do change? What fear will you have to face?

3   What will it cost you if you don't change?

4   What is your plan to maintain your restoration regarding these changes?

5   Who will you be accountable to as you pursue this commitment?

6   What are the details of this commitment? What information will you share with your accountability team when you touch base with them this week?

DEVOTIONAL

Like snow in summer or rain in harvest,
honor is not fitting for a fool.
² Like a fluttering sparrow or a darting swallow,
an undeserved curse does not come to rest.
³ A whip for the horse, a bridle for the donkey,
and a rod for the backs of fools!
⁴ Do not answer a fool according to his folly,
or you yourself will be just like him.
⁵ Answer a fool according to his folly,
or he will be wise in his own eyes.
⁶ Sending a message by the hands of a fool
is like cutting off one's feet or drinking poison.
⁷ Like the useless legs of one who is lame
is a proverb in the mouth of a fool.
⁸ Like tying a stone in a sling
is the giving of honor to a fool.

PROVERBS 26:1-8

 Read Proverbs 26.

SWORD DRILL

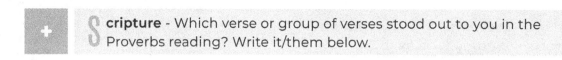

Scripture - Which verse or group of verses stood out to you in the Proverbs reading? Write it/them below.

Wait - Take a few moments now to wait on the Holy Spirit. Put aside any thoughts and worries of the day. Meditate on the Scripture. Read the verse(s) above aloud, slowly and attentively. Then pause to let it sink in. Let the Holy Spirit speak to you.

Observe - What did you notice about the verse(s) from above? Was there something that the Holy Spirit spoke to you? Write your observation below.

Request - Ask God to show you where and how the Scripture and observation apply to your life. Write the application below.

Dedicate Yourself - Looking at how the Scripture applies to you, what is one thing that needs to change? Remember, this is not necessarily about something you need to do (or stop doing). Perhaps the change is in the way you see yourself or others.

FASTER SCALE

Adapted with permission from *The Genesis Process* by Michael Dye.

- Circle the behaviors that you identify with in each section.
- Identify the most powerful behavior in each section and write it next to the corresponding heading.
- Answer the following three questions:
  1. How does it affect me? How do I feel in the moment?
  2. How does it affect the important people in my life?
  3. Why do I do this? What is the benefit for me?

RESTORATION _____

(Accepting life on God's terms, with trust, grace, mercy, vulnerability and gratitude.)
No current secrets; working to resolve problems; identifying fears and feelings; keeping commitments to meetings, prayer, family, church, people, goals, and self; being open and honest, making eye contact; increasing in relationships with God and others; true accountability.

1. _____
2. _____
3. _____

FORGETTING PRIORITIES _____

(Start believing the present circumstances and moving away from trusting God. Denial; flight; a change in what's important; how you spend your time, energy, and thoughts.)
Secrets; less time/energy for God, meetings, church; avoiding support and accountability people; superficial conversations; sarcasm; isolating; changes in goals; obsessed with relationships; breaking promises and commitments; neglecting family; preoccupation with material things, TV, computers, entertainment; procrastination; lying; overconfidence; bored; hiding money; image management; seeking to control situations and other people.

1. _____
   _____
2. _____
   _____
3. _____
   _____

ANXIETY

(A growing background noise of undefined fear; getting energy from emotions.) Worry, using profanity, being fearful; being resentful; replaying old, negative thoughts; perfectionism; judging other's motives; making goals and lists that you can't complete; mind reading; fantasy, codependent rescuing; sleep problems, trouble concentrating, seeking/creating drama; gossip; using over-the-counter medication for pain, sleep or weight control; flirting.

1. _____
   _____
2. _____
   _____
3. _____
   _____

SPEEDING UP

(Trying to outrun the anxiety which is usually the first sign of depression.) Super busy and always in a hurry (finding good reason to justify the work); workaholic; can't relax; avoiding slowing down; feeling driven; can't turn off thoughts; skipping meals; binge eating (usually at night); overspending; can't identify own feelings/needs; repetitive negative thoughts; irritable; dramatic mood swings; too much caffeine; over exercising; nervousness; difficulty being alone and/or with people; difficulty listening to others; making excuses for having to "do it all."

1. _____
   _____
2. _____
   _____
3. _____
   _____

TICKED OFF

(Getting adrenaline high on anger and aggression.) Procrastination causing crisis in money, work, and relationships; increased sarcasm; black and white (all or nothing) thinking; feeling alone; nobody understands; overreacting, road rage; constant resentments; pushing others away; increasing isolation; blaming; arguing; irrational thinking; can't take criticism; defensive; people avoiding you; needing to be right; digestive problems; headaches; obsessive (stuck) thoughts; can't forgive; feeling superior; using intimidation.

1. _____

2. _____

3. _____

EXHAUSTED _____

(Loss of physical and emotional energy; coming off the adrenaline high, and the onset of depression.) Depressed; panicked; confused; hopelessness; sleeping too much or too little; can't cope; overwhelmed; crying for "no reason"; can't think; forgetful; pessimistic; helpless; tired; numb; wanting to run; constant cravings for old coping behaviors; thinking of using sex, drugs, or alcohol; seeking old unhealthy people and places; really isolating; people angry with you; self abuse; suicidal thoughts; spontaneous crying; no goals; survival mode; not returning phone calls; missing work; irritability; no appetite.

1. _____

2. _____

3. _____

RELAPSE _____

(Returning to the place you swore you would never go again. Coping with life on your terms. You sitting in the driver's seat instead of God.) Giving up and giving in; out of control; lost in your addiction; lying to yourself and others; feeling you just can't manage without your coping behaviors, at least for now. The result is the reinforcement of shame, guilt and condemnation; and feelings of abandonment and being alone.

1. _____

2. _____

3. _____

GROUP CHECK-IN

COMPLETE 24 HOURS BEFORE GROUP

1 What is the lowest level you reached on the *FASTER Scale* this week?

2 What was the *Double Bind* you were dealing with?

3 Where are you on your *Commitment to Change* from our last meeting?

4 Have you lied to anyone this week either directly or indirectly?

5 What have you done to improve your relationship with your wife or other significant relationships this week?

CPSIA information can be obtained
at www.ICGtesting.com
Printed in the USA
BVHW010451231122
652533BV00012B/414

9 781943 291892